Praise for *My Mom My Hero*

"Lisa Hirsch has the remarkable ability to help people touched by Alzheimer's see that the disease opens as well as closes doors. With humor, compassion, and insight, her observations remind us to stay open to the unexpected gifts the experience brings. *My Mom My Hero* is filled with love and a deep appreciation for the human spirit. It's a book to return to over and over."

—Laura Stein, best-selling author

"People who are caring for a loved one with dementia or Alzheimer's face not only the monumental day-to-day tasks of caregiving but also enormous emotional turmoil brought on by the unraveling of their relationship with a person so important to their life. With grace, humor, and empathy, Lisa Hirsch shows us how to live in the moment and savor the special, even sacred times we can still create with the people we care for, no matter how difficult the circumstances. This book is a rare gift for anyone who reads it."

**—Holly Robinson, author of *Sleeping Tigers*
and *The Wishing Hill***

"Ms. Hirsch transforms her relationship with her mother through a maze of memories and imaginings brought on by Alzheimer's. We follow her story with personal hope— can we reconcile our own mother-daughter relationship with such grace and humor?"

**—Darlene Markovich, founder,
*The Missing Peace Project***

"Lisa Hirsch takes us on this wonderful journey about how her distant relationship with her mother is set aside when her mom is diagnosed with Alzheimer's. Lisa becomes energized by her mother's courage and takes on the role of core caregiver. Clearly another lesson on how love conquers all. A must read for anyone dealing with elder care."

—Pat Moffett, author of *Ice Cream in the Cupboard*

"With her cheery spirit and thoughtful reflection, Lisa Hirsch shows us how we can have meaningful relationships with loved ones suffering from Alzheimer's. *My Mom My Hero* is a light of inspiration in a world that can be dark and frustrating. To me it's a story with two heroes—mother and daughter."

—Franz Wisner, *New York Times* best-selling author of
Honeymoon with My Brother and
How the World Makes Love

My Mom
My Hero

Alzheimer's—A Mother and
Daughter's Bittersweet Journey

Lisa R. Hirsch

Logan Shawn Press

My Mom My Hero: Alzheimer's—A Mother and Daughter's Bittersweet Journey
Copyright © 2013 Lisa R. Hirsch
Published by Logan Shawn Press

DISCLAIMER
Actual people's names have all been changed to protect their privacy.

Visit the blog at www.MommyHero.blogspot.com

Book design by:
Arbor Books, Inc.
www.arborbooks.com

Printed in the United States of America

My Mom My Hero: Alzheimer's—A Mother and Daughter's Bittersweet Journey
Lisa R. Hirsch

1. Title   2. Author   3. Memoir

Library of Congress Control Number: 2013903463
ISBN: 978-0-615-77398-8

I dedicate this book to my mother,
Ruth Elian, for always loving me and
being there for me whether I knew it or not.

As Mother Teresa said,
"Not all of us can do great things.
But we can do small things with great love."

My mom has Alzheimer's. Out of her suffering with this disease, she has inspired me to write a diary of our journey together. Our relationship has blossomed into a true love affair. As a teenager I had wished for someone else to be my mother, but today I would never trade her for any other mom in the world. Each and every day she touches my heart. I'd love to share our story with you and what living with Alzheimer's is all about.

Ten percent of profits earned will be donated to Us Against Alzheimer's.

Table of Contents

Introduction

This is a story of love, dedication, discovery, and transformation. It is the story of my mother-in-law's journey into Alzheimer's and the newfound love from a daughter to her mother.

Lisa and I don't really know when the disease first started. Its effects are at first subtle and hard to discern. Looking back we can identify the first signs, but when they first appeared we were more bothered and baffled than sympathetic and caring.

This is a strange disease; impossible to treat, the sufferer slips into a world with diminished awareness and capacity. The family and caregivers go through their own journey. Starting off in ignorance, one is forced to face the reality of the disease and has the choice of denial or acceptance. There is no correct response. Each family will find their own way of coping.

Ruthie was always a cute, spunky spirit who freely expressed her opinions and doted on our son Logan. Her annual trips up from Florida were nice times to spend together, with her and Logan sharing bowls of popcorn as they watched his favorite movies. Over time, though, these trips became more problematic. She seemed less attentive and more argumentative. What had been something to look forward to became something to get through.

Once we learned Ruthie's diagnosis, my wife's response started to shift. Lisa became a more caring and concerned daughter. Her daily phone calls to her mother and the caregivers defined her involvement and response. When I got home from my work at the VA Hospital, she would tell me what had transpired. On weekends, I often sat by and listened as Lisa had the speaker phone on. I heard the love and humor that flowed back and forth. Despite the disease, Ruth had not lost her charm and quickness of thought.

I remember saying to Lisa, "You should write some of this stuff down."

Well, that's what she started to do. In a little spiral notebook, Lisa noted her mom's pithy remarks and her own emotional responses. Not long after that, she decided to start a blog. She posted her thoughts and experiences with Ruth weekly on Blogger and Facebook. Pretty soon people started to respond. It was amazing. Lisa started to receive comments and e-mails from all around the world: the United States, Canada, England, Spain, Germany, Russia, India, Israel, and many other countries. She realized what she had already known: this is a disease without borders.

Not only family members, but Alzheimer's associations, caregivers, nurses, physicians, and support group members wrote to say how she had touched their hearts, how she was speaking for all of them. They especially liked her upbeat approach, choosing to celebrate the love she still had and which had grown immeasurably. Alzheimer's can sap the energy and joy from family members, but Lisa remained energized. Any past ambivalence toward her mother had been transformed to love and devotion.

When she had a career in the fashion industry, Lisa would bemoan the fact that while I "made a difference in others lives," she only designed and sold clothes. I would reassure her that fashion, too, could make a difference in a person's life. Now Lisa is living her wish to make another kind of difference, in a meaningful and worldwide way.

Relationships are often like an equation. For Lisa and Ruth, the relationship is now stronger but also unequal. For one love grows, while for the other it fades. Regarding devotion, one gives more and one gives less. This is a true journey with many curves, hills, and valleys. What is most rewarding is seeing how my wife's connection to love and support has immeasurably been transformed. For this I, too, am grateful and rewarded.

We hope you will be touched and inspired as so many of her readers have already been. We are all in this together.

    —Bert Hirsch
      Husband
      Son-in-Law
      Program Director, Psychosocial Rehabilitation
      and Recovery Center
      Brooklyn VA Medical Center

February 20, 2011

Girl With a Curl

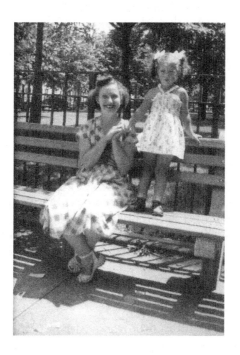

My mom is my hero today and forever. It all began many years ago when I was born in Brooklyn. I was told that at a young age, I was either singing, dancing, or shedding tears. My moods were never in between. I was either happy or I was sad.

My mom recited a special poem to me when I was a child, a poem that I will never forget. Although my mom has no memory left since she has Alzheimer's, it amazes me that she is still able to recite it.

> There was a little girl,
> Who had a little curl,
> Right in the middle of her forehead.
> When she was good,
> She was very very good,
> But when she was bad she was horrid.

More recently, I was sitting in a park and saw a little girl with blonde, curly hair playing with her mother. I watched as she hugged her mother tightly. She must have been around three years old. I wondered if I had also done that with my mom when I was that young. I have no memory of it at all, but what flashed into my head once again was the poem that she always said to me. It brought much warmth to my heart and filled me with special memories.

> There was a little girl,
> Who had a little curl,
> Right in the middle of her forehead.
> When she was good,
> She was very very good,
> But when she was bad she was horrid.

Loving the Mom
I Never Appreciated

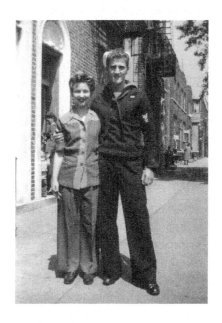

My mother, Ruth Esther Schnitzer, grew up in Brooklyn and married my father in 1942. She was blonde, pretty, and petite—just under five feet tall—and wore her hair in a pixie cut that suited her feisty personality.

Ruth's parents left Russia to move to America for a better life. Her father went to work in a sweat shop in New York's garment district, striving to give his children better opportunities than he had. With his encouragement, Ruth loved to read and learn. She continued taking college classes most of her adult life.

My mom gave birth to my brother Gil during World War II when she was just eighteen years old. She moved in with her parents when my father shipped out with the Navy. Mom worked at the military base, and my grandmother cared for my brother. When my dad got out of the service, Gil was two years old, and my grandmother and Mom were so protective that Dad could hardly have a relationship with him.

Naturally, when I was born five years later, Dad showered me with affection. I adored him as much as he adored me. He was carefree and upbeat, always telling jokes or singing show tunes. He spoiled me, and sometimes I wonder if that's why Mom was so hard on me. Maybe she resented me in some way and felt jealous.

Mom was adamant that I should make the most of myself. She ordered summer reading materials and wouldn't let me out to play until I mastered one lesson every day. I fought those lessons, especially the summer that she handed me particularly difficult assignments that turned out to be for children a grade ahead of me. I felt like I was being tortured, and I disliked reading for years afterward.

As a child and an adolescent, I built up resentments and anger toward my mother. I dreamed of a warmer, more nurturing mother to call my own. As I grew older, my feeling remained the same until my mom got Alzheimer's.

After I was married and had a child of my own, I'd get

excited whenever Mom came to visit from Florida. Then I couldn't wait until she left because all we did was argue. She'd start fights with me and say she was never coming to visit again because I was crazy. I'd tell my husband that I never wanted to see her again, but every year the same pattern repeated itself. Why? What were we getting out of it? How is it possible that I can only realize how deeply I love her now, and couldn't then?

I didn't realize how far my mother's Alzheimer's had progressed until five years ago, when I flew down to visit and experienced a terrible shock. My mother, always proud of her appearance and housekeeping, was dressed in dirty, disheveled clothing. She looked like a bag lady. When I asked if she wanted to comb her hair, Mom picked up her toothbrush and used that. She hadn't flushed the toilet. Her mirrors were so covered with dirt that it was impossible to see any reflection. Her kitchen cabinets and microwave were coated with food drippings. It was clear that she had no idea what food was in her refrigerator, if she had eaten, or how to use the microwave.

I tried to talk Mom into moving to New York. My dad had passed away several years before, and I thought she'd want to live closer to me, where I could also be able to watch over her. New York, of course is her childhood home. But she was steadfast in her determination to stay in her home in Florida where she'd been so happy with my dad. My brother and I had several discussions, and we decided that our mother needed someone to look after her.

Mom now struggles to remember the name of the man I've been married to for thirty years. She has signs posted around her apartment to remind her to do even the smallest daily routines: "Flush toilet," "Brush teeth," "Wear clothes, tops and bottoms." Will her mind soon become a blank canvas?

Life can be strange. Today my mom, whom I once argued with every day of my life, has become a delight and inspires me with her strength, courage, and joy.

Our lives go by so quickly. We don't get to pick and choose our own grand finales. We march through events that will become memories without stopping to examine them as they're happening. More days, months, years are behind us, gone before we know it. Why should I make a big deal of my mother's losing her memory when she does not? Like a child, Mom lives in the moment, and most of her moments are happy ones.

"Mom, if you could wish for anything you wanted today, what would it be?" I asked the last time I called.

"For my children to be healthy and happy!" she said with such joy in her voice.

If I could wish for anything today, I'd wish that Mom could grow old without any illnesses. Since I can't have that, I am grateful for this new way of being with her. If my mother hadn't gotten Alzheimer's, I would never have learned to love her so unconditionally. All of the qualities that once drove me away—her energy, her courage, her wisdom, her strength—now draw me to her.

Mom, I dedicate this book to you and all the other families that are struggling with this disease called Alzheimer's. My mom has truly become my hero. I love her so deeply and hope that she will never forget that as she slowly fades away.

TESTIMONIALS

Lisa,

Just wanted to send you a note to thank you for your inspirational blog. I read it last night when I needed to see another person's perspective on their relationship with their mom with Alzheimer's disease. My mom is newly diagnosed, and I am starting to come to terms with it. I am tired of feeling helpless. A lot of the information and stories shared by others are quite depressing, and to be honest, right now I need something positive. You have provided that by writing honestly about your loving acceptance of your mom and where she on her journey with Alzheimer's today. Please keep sharing your story!

—Natalie

Hello Lisa,

I just happened to stumble upon your blog today. I want you to know you are very inspiring with your story and the way you've opened up about your relationship with your mom. My mom also has Alzheimer's. She was diagnosed at the age of fifty-two. She is now fifty-six. My father and I are her full-time caregivers. I am struggling every day with trying to hold on to what little glimpses of her may show up. I truly just want to thank you for opening up and letting me in.

—Emily

Lisa,

I love reading your blog. You are so sweetly upbeat and positive. You are an inspiration to me, as you help me keep me "sunny side up."

—Randy

Just wanted to say I have been reading your blog. It feels like you are talking about my mom. So many of the things you say are what I go through every day. Twice this month she showed real excitement in seeing me. This felt good, but I knew something wasn't quite right. Then she proceeded to tell me that I was her mother and she was my daughter. I know from going through this for two years, with both parents having Alzheimer's, that you try to laugh and gently see if you can get them going on the right track. After several minutes she looked at me and said, "I am your mother"! I said, "That's right. You are my mom!" I had a very difficult relationship with my mother for the first fifty years of my life. We never got along. Since April 2010, when she suffered a stroke and a grand mal seizure, things have changed. As much as I hate this disease, I am so glad that I have had these last two years to spend with my mom. I love her so much. Thanks for blogging and listening to me.

—Cheri

Hi Lisa,

I have just found your blog about you and your mom, and it really hit home. My mum was diagnosed with Alzheimer's three years ago. I live in England and she lives in Northern Ireland, which means we have a plane journey between us. Your blog is amazing, and it feels comforting to recognize similar traits in our mums. Anyway, please keep blogging!

Kind regards,
Sara

Trading Places, or
Is Alzheimer's Catching?

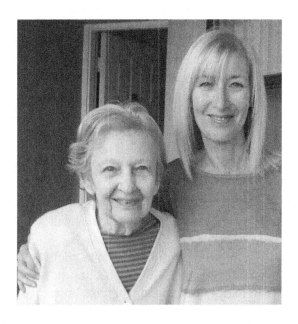

Iseemed to switch places with my mom today. I became her, and she became me. This morning she tried to help me find the mascara that I had misplaced. While on the phone with her, I was getting ready to put my eye makeup on. I can easily do that while I have her on the speaker phone. I began to move about, which is what I do from time to time. While speaking to her, I realized that

I could not find my mascara. As we continued to talk, I kept opening and closing the draws in my bathroom vanity, hoping that my makeup would reappear. I started getting upset when my mom said, "So you'll go buy new ones." I answer, "That's not the point. I always keep them in the same place, so where can they be?"

Mom told me to check my handbag by removing everything from it. After emptying my bag, I still could not find my makeup. She then told me to retrace every place where I have been. I looked in my handbag again and even the kitchen garbage. How could I have accidently thrown out my mascara? My mother Ruthie told me next to look in the clothes I wore yesterday, along with my robe, which I had already done. She wanted to know how much it would cost to replace the makeup. "Maybe thirty dollars," I said, "but Mom, that's not the point. How can they just disappear?" She then told me not to worry and reassured me that they will reappear. I started to laugh.

Did I become her or did she become me? Did we just trade places? I did not enjoy the feeling of being confused. I could not understand what had happened to my makeup that each day is always in the same place.

I've been with Mom when she goes through similar episodes and looks in her handbag for her four pairs of glasses. She seems to wander back and forth trying to find what she has misplaced. I feel lots of compassion for her as she keeps looking, not understanding what she did with them. While I understand what I am doing, I cannot help feeling confused and frustrated. How could I have lost my makeup? Where could it be? What was happening to me? Could I also be in the early stages of Alzheimer's? I certainly hope not.

After I hung up, I found my makeup, which was lying on the floor behind my toilet. Why didn't I think of looking there, before I went through garbage cans and had an anxiety attack? I called Mom back to tell her I found it. She wanted to know where, and we both began to giggle. I told her that I felt like her for a moment, and she replied, "Why? I have a good memory and I don't lose things." Sure, Mom, whatever you say.

She was still looking for her watch that she couldn't find for a year, only to later say that she never had one. We were like the blind leading the blind for a few minutes. My mom, my hero, stayed cool and calm as she suggested to me where I should look. It felt good that my mom, maybe for only a moment, could take care of me. This left me with a warm wonderful feeling, which I so badly needed to embrace.

COMMENTS

> I loved this. Went through it with my own mom and it brought back some wonderful memories.
>
> —Anonymous

≈≈≈≈

> I just happened upon this blog and post quite by accident, but I wanted to tell you what

a gift it was to read this tonight. I'm only beginning to come to terms with my mom's dementia. The grief and the fear is often too overwhelming for me to deal with the way I should, the way I want to, but I am trying hard to find my way back to my mom. I owe so much to her. I can't abandon her now.

—Angela

Hi Lisa,

What a special treat it was for me to read your blog about your sweet mom.

Alzheimer's disease and other dementia can be so cruel. My dear mom had dementia during the last year or so of her life. When Mom passed away, I moved into my parents' home to care for my dad, who also suffered from dementia; he attended an adult daycare facility during the day so that I could continue working. I was his caregiver for three and a half years when cancer took his life in 1990. I later married a wonderful gentleman who now, at age seventy-two, is showing some signs of memory loss. His mother, at the time of her death, had a form of dementia, and we are both aware of a genetic connection, although Joel hasn't been diagnosed yet. I am, at this moment, attempting to deal with feelings about caring for another loved one who may end up with this terrible condition. It is wonderful that you maintain a positive attitude during the times spent with Ruthie, both in person as well as on the phone. That will get you through the rough times and provide some lovely memories. May God bless you as you travel this path with your beautiful mom.

—Channel

Birthday Dedication
to the One I Love

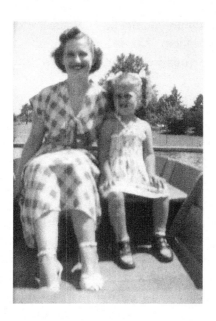

Tomorrow is my birthday. Today when I spoke to my mom, I asked her to practice her singing with me because tomorrow I would love for her to sing me the lyrics of the Happy Birthday song. We both giggled like teenage girls, as I delighted in the fact that mom is still able to remember the words.

I amusingly asked her if she could believe that she

gave birth to me so many years ago. Ruthie laughed and replied, "If you tell me that I did, then I will believe you." Mom, because of Alzheimer's, cannot even remember when I was born or how old I am. In fact, she has no idea how old she is either. Maybe that is not such a bad thing.

"Mom, would you like to guess how old I am?"

Ruthie replied, "No, I don't remember, and as long as you have your health and are alive, that is all that matters."

Okay, Mom, my post today on my blog is dedicated to the one I love. My mom, named Ruthie.

My mom gave birth to me when she was twenty-four years old. She cuddled me, fed me, and dressed me. She sent me to ballet school, gave me piano lessons, sent me to sleep-away camp, took me on vacations, and toured historic sites with me, as well as cultural events, museums, and concerts. My mom who took care of me as a young child and through my teenage years, then sent me off to college and watched as I became a bride (not once, but twice) and later as I became a mother myself.

This is the mom who watched and took care of my dad for nine long months as he was in a nursing home dying. My mom has held her head high and has shown me much strength and courage. My mom, although she suffers from Alzheimer's and macular degeneration at the age just shy of eighty-seven, never seems to complain or sound depressed. Every day when I phone, she sounds so cheerful. When I say hello, I can feel the smile on her face and laughter in her heart as she says, "Hi, sweetie."

This is my mom whom I have fallen deeply and passionately in love with the last several years.

This is the mom who gave birth to me, brought me into this world, and raised me to be a caring human being. This is the mom I want to thank. This is the mom who has become my hero.

Today with my birthday one day away, I want to thank her for all that she has done and dedicate to her all my love. Without my mom, I would not be here. Thank you, Mom. This I dedicate to you.

COMMENTS

Hi Lisa,

I saw your blog today for the first time, and it really touched me. I posted a brief note but also wanted to personally write here and thank you for writing your love story to your mom and for sharing your personal journey. It actually gave me strength and some clarity, too. My seventy-nine-year-old mother also has Alzheimer's, and my father has dementia from a severe stroke. I am the primary caregiver, since my brother lives out of state. Thanks again, as I will be following you along your journey with your mother.

—Alyce

Lisa,

You are tonic. Others talk about the challenges while you talk about the relationship. Again, you are truly tonic.

—Mary, United Kingdom

What's My Daughter's Name?

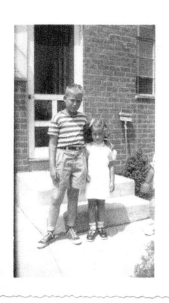

I want to stay upbeat and positive, although as I write this post, I am honestly feeling a little frightened and upset. I called my brother to share with him what our mother had said yesterday to me. Or, should I say, what she did not say. It certainly left me feeling a little bewildered and with a heavy heart.

As my mom answered the phone, I greeted her with a perky hello. "Hi, Mom, and how are you feeling today?"

She answered, "Just fine, sweetie," which immediately put a big smile on my face and much joy in my heart. I excitedly told Mom how I just met another girl named Lisa Elian. Please let me explain. Elian is my maiden name, and an unusual one at that. I did not bother to tell Mom that I met her on Facebook or that she lived in Austria, which is where my dad's father was from. Maybe we are related? I did share this part with mom.

Ruthie laughed out loud and said, "Really? That's very funny, because my name is Lisa Elian." Did I just hear my mom correctly or was I hearing things? "Mom, I thought your name was Ruth." She answered, "No, I have two names, Lisa and Ruth." "Well, Mom, then who am I?" She said, "I'm not sure who I am speaking to." Was I hearing things? Mom had just called me "sweetie," after she answered the phone.

"Mom, I'm your daughter, and my name is Lisa. Maybe you just want to call yourself Lisa because you love me so much." She laughed, and at that moment, I think she realized her confusion.

After I hung up, I tried to call my brother. He did not answer. I shared all this with my husband, and I couldn't help feeling a little shaken up. I was then left with the scary thought: What was happening to my mother?

The next day I finally reached my brother Gil. He agreed that she was getting worse. I called Mom again today, and this time I asked her if she could spell my name. Mom answered, "I don't even know your name." "Mom, not only am I your daughter, you also gave me my name. Can you guess what my name is?" First she says,

"Is it Trudy?" She then quickly says, "Lisa." *Very good, Mom*, I think, and then say, "What is your name?" Mom says, "Ruth."

Tomorrow when I call, and every day after, I will start my calls with, "Hi Mom, it's Lisa, your daughter," so my mom will hopefully be sure to remember my name.

COMMENTS

> Thank you so much for creating this profile. I have cried when reading some of the things you've posted here. My mom's Alzheimer's was discovered recently when it was already 18 on a scale of 30. She has been getting worse every few moments, while other moments she is just fine. My love and compassion have been growing. I still have more to bring out. It's been so painful seeing her like this. The acceptance has recently just begun working inside me. I love her so much and always want her to know it, because yes, it's true, she forgets that, too! I love your page because it's just what I and many others need. Thank you!
> —Stacey

Your relationship with your mom is inspirational and worthy of sharing. Thank you for doing so. You will encourage many of us who are struggling with relationships that have been affected by dementia.

—A Place for Mom

Happy Birthday, Mom

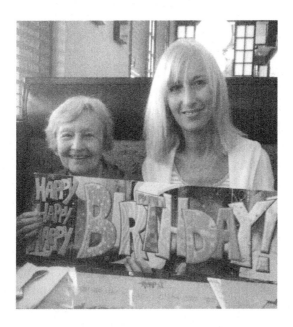

Today is August 24, 2011. It is a very special day in more ways than one. I am so excited because today my mom turns eighty-seven years young. When I shared this with Ruthie, she replied, "Eighty-seven years old. Wow, am I really that old?" "Yes, Mom." She then replied, and I quote her, "Well, at least I don't look my age." And with that, we both laughed.

Fortunately she still is filled with much spunk and energy. I do think that she looks her age, yet I will certainly not say so. Why would I spoil her day? If Ruthie thinks she looks young, that's all that matters. You see, my mom's eyesight is failing, because she also has macular degeneration. This is something that she never mentions nor complains about.

Besides it being her birthday, there are also threats that Hurricane Irene is close to Florida's shores. When I spoke with Mom's caregiver Elaine, she shared with me that she was going to get a cake and come back to Mom's at the same time that my brother would be arriving. She also reassured me that if the hurricane was going to be threatening in anyway, she would stay over at my mom's house. Elaine so caringly did not want Mom to be all alone.

Elaine is so kind and thoughtful for offering this. She and her daughter Trudy take such wonderful care of my mom. We are very fortunate to have each of them.

Elaine put Mom back on the telephone, and I shared with her what Elaine had just told me. Mom repeated everything that I said right back to Elaine. I was amused by this, and I told her that Elaine was so nice to her because she was so sweet. We both giggled, and sure enough, she repeated what I just said, once again to Elaine.

I then heard Mom say, "Lisa, you are a doll, and I love you so much." "Mom, you're going to make me cry." She answered, "Please don't cry." "Mom, they would be tears of joy." After we hung up, my heart felt like it could explode with how much love I felt for her.

It's hard to believe that before my mom got Alzheimer's there were moments when we fought and did not get along. Sometimes, for a quick second, I did not care if we saw each other again. Today all I want to do is hold on to her, love her, and cherish every second that she still knows my name and who I am. Ruthie, my mom, now is to me one special lady.

So Mom, I dedicate to you all my love and wish that all my writings about you and our relationship are able to touch other people, just like you have touched me. I would also want to wish you a very special birthday and send you all my love, sealed with a kiss.

xoxo
Lisa

COMMENTS

Hi Lisa,

I love your blog. My mom too suffers with Alzheimer's. I recently went to my first walk to end Alzheimer's, and the emotions I felt were none that I would have expected. It was like a burden was lifted off of me, because for the first time I felt, "Hey, our family is not the only one going through this journey!" (Even though, of course, I knew realistically we were not.) It was just that feeling of actually physically seeing others going through the same journey. It was almost like a relief, which is a weird feeling because you do not wish this disease on anyone. But, for a lack of a better word, that is exactly how I felt. Reading your blogs has also made feel I am not alone! I am the only girl in a family with three boys, whom by the way I love dearly, but who are absolutely no help when it comes to the care of my mother. (LOL!)

My dad is my mom's primary caregiver, and I am her secondary caregiver. I only live two hours from my parents' home and can go there quite often to assist my dad with her care. I hate hate hate this disease, but I have fallen in love with my "other" mom. I have learned to let go of the person that was and to embrace the person that is. This disease has definitely shown me the true meaning of love. I will keep you in my thoughts and prayers as we go through this journey with our moms. Thanks again for sharing your thoughts!

—Kassey

Feelings,
Oh So Many Feelings

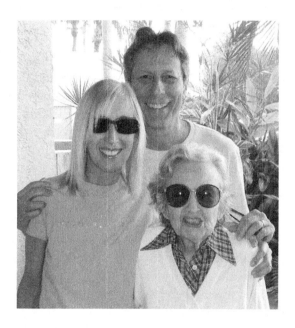

"Mom, do you know your mother?" "No Lisa, I do not remember her." "Mom, who are you to me?" My mom then answered, "I am your good friend," as she gave me a kiss on the top of my head as she exited the room. My heart sank for a moment, and when she came back I responded with, "Mom, I love you so much." She then said, "I love you also." I asked, "As your daughter?" "Yes, Lisa, as my daughter, and my friend."

This was pretty much how my visit with Mom was this trip. It made me realize that her Alzheimer's was progressing. I was so grateful that my husband had come with me and that we were not staying at her home. I was able to spend six days with her, and when I left fortunately I had my husband's love and support to help me cope with my mom's condition.

While I was in one room, my husband in another, and my mom in another, my husband heard my mom say, "Is anyone here, is anyone here?" We answered, and she then said, "Someone please come here. I'm very lonesome."

Monday, the day before we left to go back home, my mom seemed listless. She had no energy, nor did she want to do anything. Mom was not interested in anything as simple as even getting or giving hugs. As I sat at the airport the next day, waiting to return home, I felt my eyes filling up with tears. My heart felt quite heavy, and I experienced sadness as I wondered what might lie ahead.

The next day when I phoned, Mom wanted to know when I would be coming to see her. Although I had just left, she had no memory of my having been there. It's ironic—I get upset when I see her, and I get even sadder when I cannot see her.

I wonder why after every trip visiting her I feel like I'm getting sick. I return feeling trapped and perhaps helpless. I feel helpless in the sense that there is nothing that I could possibly do to help my mom. Her whole life and existence has disappeared like it never existed. The thought that this disease can do this to anyone boggles my mind. Since it is my mom, it also breaks my heart in two.

I want to hold her and be able to protect her, a feeling that I share for my own child. Our roles have reversed, although I still get glimpses of my "real" mom. There are parts of her at moments that are still able to shine. Either way for me, there is a pang that still remains in my heart.

On Thursday my spirits finally lifted after I spoke to her. My mom was having a great day. She was alert, sharp, and sounding happy. It's amazing how much lighter I became. I told her that she was my favorite mom. We both giggled as she then said to me, "You're lucky because I'm your only mom." It was only three days ago that Mom thought she was my friend and not my mother. I shared with her that she sounded so happy, and she responded that she is always happy. This was a blessing that I loved to hear.

I know that this may not last, yet I loved our conversation. I feel happy and excited, and I rejoice in the happiness that today she was able to express. It's amazing from one day to the next how she can change. Surely what a difference a day can make.

COMMENTS

> Thanks for continuing to write and share, Lisa. It's a journey you and your mother are on. Many others are on the same journey relate to what you share. Merry Christmas!
> —Martha

I really enjoy your blog. I hope you will find solace in keeping this journal. I appreciate reading about how much you love her!

—Sally

I stumbled upon your blog from Caring-bridge on Facebook. As a med aide/caregiver in a memory care unit, I have the honor to take care of some wonderful people who become like family to me. Although we "see" what families are dealing with, we never truly "see" it. The words you write really touched my core. To get a glimpse of your feelings and struggles and happy times with your momma is a blessing. Bless you and your mom!

—Christine

I also can relate to your posting. My mother cannot communicate anymore, but I feel that visiting is so important at any stage of dementia. Even though she does not recognize me anymore, I know holding her hand and being there makes a difference. I grab what I can and make this a "good day" experience no matter how little a ray of sunshine beams down into the grey clouds of this disease. I wish you and your mom many more good days. Dementia is so hard.

—Elissa

Lisa,

Her whole life and existence will never "disappear" because she has a daughter like you, who will always remember and cherish the "real" mom. Sometimes I have to struggle to remember my "real" dad, and not the man who merely existed before his passing. But then I look at great pictures of him, like the ones that you've posted here of your sweet mom, and the good memories come flooding back. Best wishes to you and your family. Keep on keeping on. Yes, each day really does make a difference.

—Anonymous

Lisa,

I can completely understand all of the different feelings that we go through while on this journey with our loved ones. My mom is in the very late stages, is now having issues swallowing her food, and cannot communicate what she needs or wants, so I am her voice. This is a very horrible process to have to watch someone you love go through. But, even at this stage, I watch mama have really good days where I know she is aware that I am there. Then there are the days where she just stares off into space and I practically have to get in her face to look at her. I lost my daddy just four short years ago to stage 4 colon cancer and am not ready for my mama to go be with him. Mama and I have always had a close relationship, but this has bonded us that much closer, if that was even possible. I'm sorry if my comment has upset anyone in any way. I am just needing to reach out to as many people as I can. Hug your mom and tell her you love her as much as you possibly can. Make as many memories from this journey as possible. I hope you had a Merry Christmas and will have a Happy New Year!

—Becca

Is This a Dream?

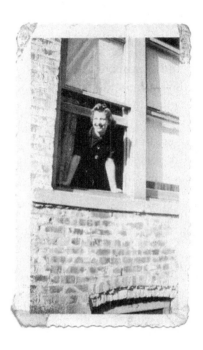

I awoke today to a rather upsetting dream, which made me think immediately of my mom. It was of a woman lying in what looked like a hospital bed, with no movement as if she were almost dead. To me the image was of my mom, and it left me feeling quite sad and empty.

I'd like to go back a few days from today and explain what has transpired with my mom. We had a magical conversation on the telephone the other day. She listened carefully as I read her a section of my blog/book about her childhood. Mom was delighted and remembered where she was born, where she grew up, her parents, her dear friend Jeanie, and her love of reading books. With enthusiasm she made comments as I read to her. I hung up the phone and was left with one big wow! This was truly amazing and a moment that I would not forget.

The next day Mom still sounded good, and I asked her if she was going to her clubhouse. Mom said to me, "No, I am not going to the clubhouse. I'm too busy." I laughed and joked around with her about what could she be so busy with. "Mom, are you going to work, or are you so busy cooking dinner?" She quickly answered no to both.

I was at the moment thrilled that Mom was able to remember that where she lived had a clubhouse. Up to then for several years, she had claimed that there was no clubhouse, which at one time was a place she had enjoyed visiting.

The following day when I called in the morning, my mom was hallucinating. I could not believe what I was hearing her say. She insisted that she wanted to go to her house and that the place she now was in was not her home. You see, Mom had lived in her home for twenty-three years. It was a place that she had shared with my dad, a home that she said she would never leave. Today this was not what she was saying. I wanted to hang up the phone and run right over to her. This is impossible since we live in different states. I felt so frightened. How could any of this be happening, when only yesterday Mom was doing so great?

I knew that my brother was visiting her today, so I hung up and I called him immediately. He arrived at Mom's around 2:00 p.m., and hours later she was still hallucinating. The second my brother arrived, Mom insisted that they leave, which is something she never wants to do. She told my brother that she lived with her parents and that she wanted to go home and be with them. My brother told her that her parents were no longer alive, and once again she insisted that they were.

My brother decided since she was hallucinating for so many hours, that he should bring her to the hospital. Something had to be terribly wrong. They admitted my mom and found that she had a urinary tract infection and put her on an antibiotic. (I have since learned that this can be common in women who have dementia— something my brother and I were not aware of.)

The second day in the hospital, Mom was speaking to me on the phone like she was on speed. She had sounded the same way as the day she was hallucinating. The only difference was she was now in the hospital, which left me feeling a little more secure.

This morning when I spoke to her, she sounded much better. I told her how much I missed her, and my mom then said, "Can you come over when I get home?" "I'd love to but I cannot get there immediately." She then said, "Lisa when was the last time you visited me?" My heart sank as I answered, "I was at your home four weeks ago." She then said, "You're not a good daughter. That was a long time ago."

"Mom, I live in New York and you live in Florida. I cannot just run over." With such clarity she answered, "Oh, I forgot that you live in New York." "Mom would you like to move back to New York so we can be together?" She then said, "Not really. I lived there for so many years and being in Florida is now like a vacation for me." *Some vacation*, I said to myself.

I shared with my brother this morning that somehow I felt that I might have been responsible for her craziness. I went on to say that I had just read to Mom about her childhood, and maybe somehow it sparked a memory for her, a memory like a dream that stayed imbedded in her mind.

I might have reawakened for her memories of long ago that have been lost, for her strong desire to go back home and be with her parents. Was my mom scared while she seemed to be hallucinating? Or was she perhaps at peace, feeling the security and warmth of her childhood and the love of her parents? Was Mom awake walking through her dream? We all have had dreams that have felt so real, warm, and comforting, that we don't want to wake up from them. Could this be what had happened to her?

For the moment, my mom seems a little better. I can hardly express how good it feels. It gives me glimmers of hope that I know will absolutely not last. I am trying to stay optimistic and appreciate the time we still have together. I do not know how long this will last. I love my mom dearly, and she still carries with her so much strength and courage. My mom continues to inspire me each day, and for this my mom remains my hero.

COMMENTS

I enjoyed reading your post about your mom. Those confusing days are difficult to watch, and those moments of clarity are what we hang on to. I can tell you love your mom very much. Take care.

—Lillian

This brought back memories for me. I just lost my mom—August 14, 2011. She had Alzheimer's. I had really lost her years before. Alzheimer's is such a sad disease. My hope is that her world was safe and secure with warm memories and not a scary, lonely place for her. Spend as much time as you can with your mom, and just love her.

—Patricia

Lisa,

I am a daughter that also has a mom suffering with a dementia-related disease. I couldn't help noticing some similarities between your mom's condition and my mom's. Have her doctors done any checking into dementia with Lewy bodies? I mention this because this is the latest diagnosis my mom has been given. Lewy bodies is a fairly rare condition that is very hard to diagnose. It is a condition where a certain protein collects around cells in the brain and block "neurons" from getting through. It causes a lot of hallucinations, dreams that they are actually living out, and many other things. I only mention this because it might be something that has been overlooked. This is fairly new condition and has only been known about mostly since 2008. It is named after the doctor who discovered it. If you go online and type in "Lewy bodies," you will get a great amount of information about this. They have yet to call it a disease as the only firm diagnosis can come with an autopsy. The patient is diagnosed through a series of questions and background information given by family and staff at the facility where patients are living. By having this diagnosis for our mom, it has helped us to understand her and where she is in her mind, and why. They need a totally different way to be looked after and approached. I hope this will be of some help to you and to perhaps others who do not really understand why their parent is having multi-delusional thoughts, etc. This may not be something that your mom has, but I felt it might be something to have looked into. We only found this by having our mom seen by a geriatric psychologist. He is a wonderful and very young doctor that has just come through much studying of Lewy bodies. I will keep you, your mom, and your family in my prayers. Thanks for sharing your stories—they have helped me to not feel so alone. It's very hard to see our moms this way. Be encouraged.

—Joyce

Is My Cup Half Empty or Half Full?

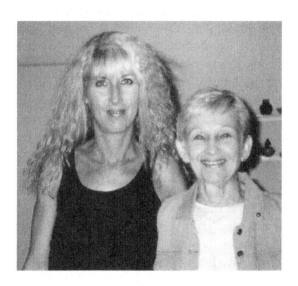

I have been walking around with a heavy heart ever since my mom was hallucinating and ended up in a hospital. This was my awakening that my mom might be ready to go into a nursing home. The thought left me feeling so sad and lonely. My feelings left me filled with much fear. How could I ever do this to her? What will she say, and how will she feel? How could I even possibly think of it?

Was I about to do the right thing? Was this best for my mom?

My mom has expressed many times that she wanted to stay in her home till she dies. I seem to remember that I had promised her that she could always remain in her home. Should I wait a couple of months, which only would be prolonging the inevitable? Maybe she could bounce back. Should I live in hope?

All this left me with many memories of my mom and dad and how quickly our lives go by. We sit, we plan, and we do not know if we'll even be around to fulfill our dreams. Lately, I have been awakening most mornings to dreams that are still as vivid after I rise from my sleep. Before this episode I was enjoying my mom completely.

I guess one could say that I looked upon the situation with that my cup was half full, not half empty. Several years ago, after I learned that my mom had Alzheimer's, I made a clear decision to cherish every second that we had left, especially since I still had the opportunity to share them with her.

Today when I called Mom, I was able to have such a fun, uplifting conversation. It lifted my spirits and left me feeling so much lighter. She told me that I had seven sisters and two brothers. The true facts are that my mom has only one daughter, which is me, and only one son. For me I was happy to play along with her, as we both giggled like teenage girls.

Mom does not remember what is true, and to me this no longer makes a difference. At this point it does not matter. I guess what I need, or so badly want, is to delight in these cute and humorous conversations whether they make sense or not.

What I have realized is that when my mom is sounding so great she might be in "la la land." When I catch her sounding a little down, she may be somewhere in her mind, wondering what is happening to her.

I cannot change or take away Alzheimer's from my mom, yet I can laugh with her and enjoy the moments that we have left. And guess what? Out of my mom's seven daughters, I'm still her favorite one. Lucky, lucky me!

So I wonder, is it better to have my cup half full or half empty? There is nothing I can change other than how I hold everything. I am grateful for all that we still have left, and cannot think about all that is lost. For this my cup will remain half full.

COMMENTS

Your story touched me deeply, I lost my mom to Alzheimer's last July, it's been a long and hard journey watching her forget who she is and who her children and grandchildren are, and watching her body slowly break down then finally losing her. My thoughts and prayers are with you and your family. Treasure your memories.

—Nanette

Be grateful for the cup. I lost Mom three years ago (it seems like yesterday) yet I hear her talking to me today. I cry from the pain of remembering but laugh at what was and keep moving forward

—Beth

Lisa,

What a gift you give us by sharing your story and love for your mother! Your story is so touching and I hope it will help others to focus on those moments of joy and life's little blessings. What a difference we can make in the world when we see the cup as half full. And I am so glad you are the favorite of the seven daughters! LOL

—Samantha

My mom died when I was eleven and my dad when I was twenty-one. I have never had to deal with aging parents. I guess I have to see your cup as half full. I know it must be difficult. You also have to keep her safe too.

I have told my children that I don't really want to go to a nursing home, but if it comes to that point I will trust them to make the right decision. I don't want to be a problem for them. Your mother sounds like she would feel the same way.

I hope you won't be too hard on yourself if you have to put her in a nursing home. Just enjoy the time you have as you are doing. Good luck to you and take care.

—Denise

Lisa,

I was very touched by your tribute to your mother. I must say the story sounds familiar in many ways. However, my mother lost her fight against this disease this month. I am torn between feeling relief that her suffering has ended and the fact that my mother has really died. I spent so much time and energy caring for her for the past few years that I am feeling a little lost right now. I have channeled my energy into raising funds and awareness for the Alzheimer's Association. However, I still find myself thinking of all the things Mom might need from me. I want to comment on the "you are her favorite daughter" thing you mentioned. How sweet! My mother has three children, two boys and me. The last year of her life I became like a sister to her. She was an only child, so that was a strange concept. However, if she got mad, she remembered I was her daughter! The very last month of her life, she seemed to think I was her daughter most of time. I treasured that. It was a small thing, but as you are aware, all the emotion and difficulties you survive when you have or care for someone with this disease make each little shining moment important. Keep up the good work—awareness is an extremely important tool in this fight against Alzheimer's. Good luck and God bless.

—Lena

A Day Filled With Sunshine

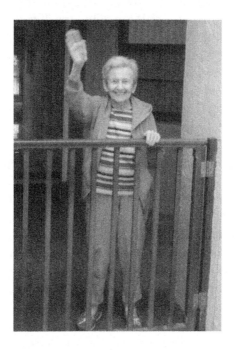

Today was a really good day for my mom, as were the last several days. My heart seems to go up and down with lightness and heaviness depending how she is doing each day. I know this has to be a normal response and I do not question it. I just know that this is how it is ever since my Ruthie became ill with Alzheimer's.

Fortunately for us, Mom still has enough good

moments for me to have a smile on my face and to delight in our daily phone calls. Just today after we sang several songs that neither of us remembered the words to, I said, "Mom, are you my sweetheart," My Ruthie answered with, "No, how could we be? We're both girls. If you were not a girl, then I could call you sweetheart." We both giggled, and at that moment I think even Mom understood how silly our conversation was. I become overjoyed just hearing the sound of her laughter.

The next part of what I'm about to share was at a moment that my heart felt quite heavy.

As I sat in the waiting room for a tour of another nursing home for my mom, I was left in deep thought and feeling rather sad. I have seen the dementia floors in several nursing homes only to keep feeling that my mom was not ready for this. Although Mom's illness will progress, I know that she has some life left in her. Bringing her to one of these places will probably upset her, and the thought of it seems to sicken me.

My husband has been touring these facilities with me, and we are sadly starting to speak about our own mortality and what might lie ahead for us. I'm sure that if my mom could reason and truly understand what her illness will be doing to her as it progresses, she'd probably wish deep in her heart to be able to say goodbye.

Mom on most days seems happy, yet she has no idea what day or year it is. She doesn't knows where she lives, nor can she remember most of the events in her life. I've often described her mind like a blank canvas. It is amazing that Alzheimer's can just remove one's life, as if it never existed. She has no idea what is happening in the world (which may not be such a bad thing). Although my mom does not remember that I just called or visited her, I know that she can still feel all the love I have for her.

Life can be great and life can be wonderful. Life can also be cruel and life can be hard. None of us know what lies ahead, so we must truly be happy and thankful for each new day that we have. Each and every day is truly a gift. I know deep in my heart that my mom only wishes for me a day filled with sunshine.

COMMENTS

I've been reading your blog for quite some time now. I can't remember how I stumbled upon it, but I am the primary caregiver to my eighty-five-year-old mother who also has Alzheimer's. Your blog touches me very much as our moms are similar in many ways. My mom is petite, a fiery redhead, who dances every chance she can get. Even her recent onset of hallucinations mirrors part of your journey as well. I know it has to be so difficult to think about having to move your mom into a nursing home. I know I will dread it when the time comes for me. Thanks for sharing your walk.

—Anonymous

Bless you for such a beautiful story of love, courage, and faithfulness. I care for my ninety-one-year-old father who also has Alzheimer's. Some days he cannot remember much of his life or who he is, but I do. No one in a facility would know my father's history. A caregiver in a facility would not know he was born into a fifteen-member family, raised on a farm with ten brothers and three sisters, that he was married for sixty-three years to my mother, that his beloved son, a police officer, is in heaven, or that when he says I love you, he really means it. As you noted with your mother, I know if my father had any comprehension of his true status, he would have wanted leave this life long ago. I pray daily for a cure for this most heart-wrenching and debilitating disease.

—Anonymous

Treasure every moment. I lost my mom to Alzheimer's on March 22, 2011, at 3:43 a.m. We nursed Mom at home. She stayed in a nursing home for about six weeks while a package of care was put into place. That was the most traumatizing thing for us to do as a family. Only now am I realizing just how brave my beautiful mother was as the last three years of her life were spent in bed. I don't know how she had the strength, but I do know she always kept her dignity especially when caregivers called to wash her. We always say now, "It's like a long goodbye," but the things Mom went through were unbelievable. I'm just glad that as a family we could be with her. I treasured every moment, even down to changing her pad, to feeding her, to washing her hair. If I could just walk one mile in her shoes, then I will happy. I feel so blessed that I am her daughter and my world has certainly changed now she's gone. I miss her so very much.

—Margie

Little Things Can Mean A Lot

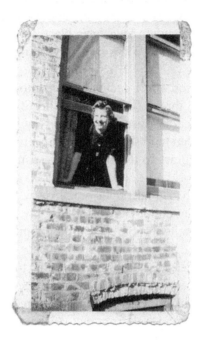

My mom grew up with an enormous thirst for learning and a true love for books. Every summer her parents took her to the country, where she would spend hours reading under a tree. I remember when as I was a child, how she delighted in sharing this experience with me. She loved words as much as she loved reading. One of her favorite books to share was *Gone With the*

Wind. Through my childhood years, she always encouraged me to read.

In 1924 when Mom was born and later in her teenage years, there was no such thing as a television. I think that her mind and love of reading made it possible for her to imagine what it might have been like to travel the world. She had a thirst to keep learning, something she took well into her aging years.

My husband and I decided to see a tour of the New York Public Library (located on 42nd Street and Fifth Avenue). It is a treasured New York City landmark that we had not been to in several years. It is probably rated as the greatest library in the United States, and ranked very high in the world. The collection of books and the beauty of this institute can take one's breath away.

As a young child, I did not share my mom's love of literature. I excitedly shared with her about my planned trip to visit the library, which she had very little response to. She did at least say, "Oh, are you going to buy a book?" Somehow, Mom was able to connect the dots to what a library might be. Her love of literature, reading, and words are now sadly all forgotten. Alzheimer's has taken that part of her world from her.

Yet since her vocabulary was one of her strengths, she still can spell almost immediately any word that I ask of her. With macular degeneration and no concentration or memory, my mother finds reading to be an impossible task for her, although her spelling skills completely amaze me.

I tried to lighten the conversation, probably more for

myself than her, and shared with her that maybe one day "our book" will appear on the shelves of the library. Mom answered with, "Maybe one day, one never knows."

I smiled to myself, because somewhere as my mom slips away, there always seems to be some shimmer of light, as words of reason still flow from her.

This may not seem like a miracle for most people, yet for someone who has had Alzheimer's for at least seven years, my mom seems to be holding on. Of course, not in many ways, yet the ways that are left for me are still so dear to my heart.

Each day that is left, I get to love my mom some more. Each day that I hear her say to her caregiver when I phone, "Oh, my daughter's on the phone," means more to me than words can ever say. So to my mom, who has become my best friend, I will also say, "Little things can mean a lot." Thanks, Mom, for being who you are.

COMMENTS

My mother suffered with this dreaded disease for at least fourteen years before she left this world. Alzheimer's is horrible and to watch a loved one go through it is truly life changing. I am sorry you are going through this. My mother died in 2005, and I am happy that she is now no longer suffering. Much love to you and your mother. Enjoy every coherent moment.

—Katrina

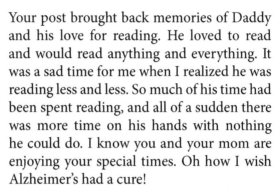

Your post brought back memories of Daddy and his love for reading. He loved to read and would read anything and everything. It was a sad time for me when I realized he was reading less and less. So much of his time had been spent reading, and all of a sudden there was more time on his hands with nothing he could do. I know you and your mom are enjoying your special times. Oh how I wish Alzheimer's had a cure!

Hugs,
Dorothy

Is This a Dream or a Nightmare?

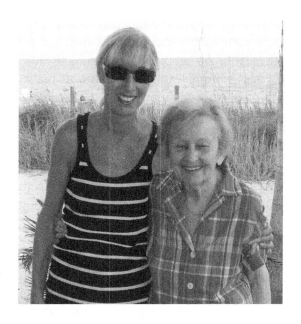

On Saturday around 10:30 in the morning I received a phone call from Elaine, my mom's caregiver. Elaine phoned to tell me that since she could not reach my brother, she would like permission to take my mother with her daughter Trudy and her grandson to the beach.

My answer was that I thought it was a lovely idea. I shared with Elaine how my mom used to love to go to the beach. I explained to Elaine that I thought it would be quite difficult for my mom to actually walk on the beach and have the hot sun beating on her. I reminded her that because of Mom's macular degeneration, the bright sun and the reflection of the water would blind her vision. I was enormously happy that Mom would be getting out and had total trust in Elaine and Trudy.

That was the last time in two days that I had any contact with my mom or her caregivers. I speak to mom every day. After not being able to reach anyone, no matter what time I tried or whose number I called, by early evening on Sunday I started to feel concerned and frightened.

On Sunday I was with my son during the day, so I was a little preoccupied and had not tried to reach anyone. I now wondered that if my mom was in a hospital. Certainly my brother or Elaine would have contacted me. Could all the phone circuits be out of order in Florida? I knew that was highly unlikely.

Finally that evening my brother called me back around 9:00 p.m. and reassured me that he had spoken to mom around 12:30 that day. He agreed with me that I had a reason to be upset, for neither Elaine nor Trudy answered their cell phones or called me back after leaving several voice mails. They split the twelve-hour shift of taking care of her, so where were they?

My mom's phone just rang and rang, and all I was left with was total silence.

I tried again between 8:00 p.m. and 8:30 p.m. when my mom is ready for bed. Still at this time her telephone just continuously rang. Where could she be? I felt so helpless and there was absolutely nothing I could do.

As I went to bed, I had a thought of what it might feel like when I would no longer be able to speak to her. There was an overwhelming emptiness that I felt inside me.

When I finally fell asleep that night, I had a dream about her. It was a lovely dream. My mom was by a beach and she seemed to have come back to life. She was changing her clothes and having conversations with other people, not exactly as my mom used to be, yet she seemed free of Alzheimer's. My mom appeared to be whole. The dream was so surreal. Yet when I awoke the feelings of heaviness were still with me.

Was it the fears of knowing that one day, even if my mom is still alive, I may not be able to speak to her? That I may not hear the sound of her voice? Or was it a deeper fear, that one day my mom would be gone? I have so many feelings, although on most days I seem to be able to stay in the moment. The moment is truly all that I have.

Was I upset because I could not speak to my mom, or was I upset for the unknown? Did I awake to a dream, or was it a nightmare, disguised in its own reality? As I speak to other adult children whose parents have Alzheimer's, this seems to be a similar fear. We sit, we wait, we watch as our parents slowly disappear from this world.

COMMENTS

> I can't have a conversation with my mom anymore, so I have to see her in person. When I can't visit for a few days in a row I get nervous—even though I know the nursing home

staff would call me if anything was wrong. I'm being a worried mom to my mother!

—Lindsay

It's a long goodbye, and we know what's down the road for us. It's not easy. It's scary knowing that our moms will forget us. We aren't there yet with our mom, and it makes me sad to know that that's going to happen eventually. I cling to everything she says and take notes because it makes me feel more connected to her.

—Elizabeth

I think that my stepfather has hit bottom with his Alzheimer's dilemma. I think he has lost some hearing at almost ninety-four. He is going to see a doctor this week to check on his mental facilities. This is wearing my mother out. She is ninety-one with macular degeneration. She has three caretakers waiting on them both. At least Al is taken each morning to an adult care center for a few hours. Lisa, it is always good to hear from you since your mother is alert and going through some of these problems. Take care.

—Anonymous

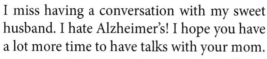

I miss having a conversation with my sweet husband. I hate Alzheimer's! I hope you have a lot more time to have talks with your mom.

—Dotty

I can still speak with my mother but it's not the same as it used to be before her dementia. Usually speaking with my mother is not a pleasant experience either. She is usually angry that she is so confused and angry with my father. I miss my "real" mom.

—Annette

You are an inspiration, Lisa. Keep the blogs coming. I am a nurse who works with Alzheimer's patients and have done so for the past thirty years, and you inspire me. Please add me as a friend so I can carry on reading your blogs.

—Grace

Feelings of My Mom

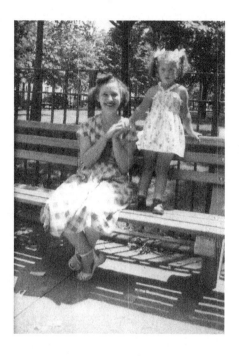

This week I had committed to volunteering at a nursing home that has one floor filled only with people who suffer from dementia. I questioned myself why I was doing this, and had thoughts of cancelling. I did not truly understand why I would place myself in an atmosphere that would only bring up my feelings about my own mother who suffers from Alzheimer's. Yet I felt that since I made the commitment, I needed to live up to it, and at least go this one time.

As I approached the building. I felt heaviness. I took a deep breath as I proceeded to go inside. I would be assisting the gentleman who comes once a week to play the piano and sing to the patients. I know how much joy singing brings to my mom, and I thought that it would be giving back to perhaps bring some joy into other people lives.

As I sang along, I was touched by a lovely lady who sat directly next to the piano player. I was told that she did not speak anymore, yet each week she came to hear him sing. I witnessed her starting to come alive and watched as the melody came out of her lips. Our eyes connected as I sang the melodies. I smiled at her, and her lips seemed to smile back. She reminded me of my mom, as my eyes slowly filled with tears. I wondered if there was anything she might have been feeling.

I thought about my own mother and wondered what at moments did she feel? These are feelings that she can no longer express, because the moment after she may think them, they just seem to vanish. Although today Mom did ask when I would be coming to see her and expressed how very much she missed me.

This sweet lady I met briefly this week deeply touched me. I had this warm feeling of wanting to take her in my arms, as I so often wish to do with my own mother. Then I wanted to tell her not to worry, that everything will be okay. I realized that one day, and I do not know when, this could be my own mom. One day her Alzheimer's will eventually win and rob her of all that she still has left.

Just as I was leaving, this sweet lady whispered to me

thank you, and we both smiled. I gently kissed her on her cheek, and once again tears for my mom swelled in my eyes.

Leaving to go home, I had such a yearning to be able to see my mother and to hold her and touch her. I shared this with my husband later that evening. For the rest of the night and into the next morning, I had an overwhelming sadness. I wondered what my mom and this lady were doing at this very moment.

Maybe deep down what I really want is for my mom to be able to hold me and squeeze me and tell me that everything will be all right. Perhaps, like the picture, I just want to be that little girl again and have my mom take care of me. As we know life does not go backwards and my wanting to be protected and cuddled by her can no longer happen. So as each day goes by, I can hold on to all that we have left and remember all the special moments of my childhood.

COMMENTS

> How lovely. What else could anyone say? Keep up the singing. It brings so much happiness to dementia clients.
>
> —Anonymous

> Wow. This really hits home for me. Thank you so much for sharing.
>
> —Anonymous

Wow! How beautifully written and how touching. I can certainly relate to this!

—Anonymous

Can't hold back the tears.

—Anonymous

I am crying my eyes out right now. We think my mother has this. My grandmother had it, and so did her brother and three sisters.

—Anonymous

A beautiful story. Thank you for sharing.

—Anonymous

Those Special Moments

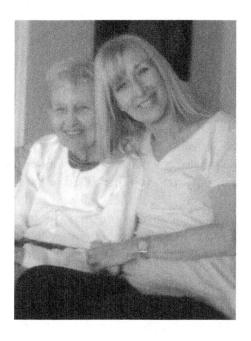

My mom has been doing great the last couple of weeks. Will it last? Who knows, and for how long? It doesn't matter. I just hold on tightly to all the love that she fills my heart with and all the smiles she adds to my face.

Today she started to speak to me in Yiddish. I think I recall that my grandfather spoke a little of it when I was young. Although he came here as a child from Europe, he learned to speak perfect English. My mom sounded great, and I was teasing her about her "new" language. I requested some lessons from her, for as a child I never heard Mom speak Yiddish.

As I hung up the phone, I laughed and was totally amazed. My mom, who cannot remember what she ate for breakfast, is now easily speaking in another language to me. Who knows where this came from? I immediately called my brother and shared it with him. His response was, "Are you serious? Mom's speaking Yiddish?" I answered, "I sure am."

Just the other day I shared with my mom something I had recently written about her. I told her the title: "My Very Special Mom." She thanked me and said that it was quite a compliment to her and that she felt honored. "Mom, if I didn't mean it I would not say it." As we both laughed, she said that it was still very sweet of me to say these things.

To keep Mom's mind stimulated, I often spell with her. I asked her to spell "compliment." Mom spelled it correctly. I then asked her to spell several other words, which she also spelled correctly. Then out of the blue, my mom said, "I don't want to spell anymore." "Why?" I inquired. She replied with that she was in bed and didn't care if she spelled or not.

"Mom, it's eleven o'clock a.m. Why are you in bed?" As if I were hearing a young child, my mom said she did not know that it was so early and asked me what she should do. "Mom, are you tired?" She answered that she didn't know. She suddenly went from spelling and sounding so sharp to now sounding like a lost child.

I once again am left with this overwhelming feeling of how I just want to hold her in my arms and to cradle her like a child. I want to have her near me, to tell her not to be afraid and that everything will be fine. Yet I know this is not how it will be.

Is it my mom that I want to hold, or is it the fears that lie deep within me? These feelings came to me from my heart, not from my head. At moments they can scare me, and at other times I forget about my mom's illness and am able to just love the special moments that we still can share.

There seems to be so much more attention to Alzheimer's lately. I have listened and read in much detail about different findings, and the optimistic feelings by neuroscientists who believe that there will be a major breakthrough within fifteen to twenty years. This will not help my mom or the millions of people around the world who now suffer from this disease. It probably would not even help me if I were to get Alzheimer's. Yet I can only imagine and pray for a world free of this disease.

This truly is a disease that only the families that are stricken with can understand. A disease that somehow can wipe away a whole person's life as if it never existed, leaving them with absolutely nothing.

So for now my mom and I still get to sing and laugh, and I get to love her completely. She can still put a smile on my face and joy in my heart. What we now can share are very special moments that I will always treasure.

COMMENTS

Hi Lisa,

I love reading your blogs. My mom also has Alzheimer's and seems to be at the same stage as your mom. My dad passed away last year, and it was only then how I realized how bad my mom was, as my dad use to cover for her. This disease is frightening, and I sometimes feel I lost both my parents last year. Mom doesn't believe that Dad has passed, and although she is in wonderful assisted living in South Africa, she constantly sits at the window waiting for his return. I visit two to three times a week, yet it breaks my heart to see her slipping away. Your blogs are dear to my heart, as I feel that there is someone out there, experiencing the same things as my family and I are currently experiencing. You are not alone. Take care.

—Cher

Wow, isn't it amazing and wonderful that your mom can still spell and also speak Yiddish. Alzheimer's is such an awful thief, robbing the person's memories, and then it's so wonderful when we get those surprise memories.

Hugs,
Dale

Lisa,

This is a beautiful tribute to your mom. What a special relationship you have with her. My mom is in the late stages of Alzheimer's disease and we just placed her on hospice. This disease is so horrific and devastating.

Best,
Sally Anne

Like a Miracle

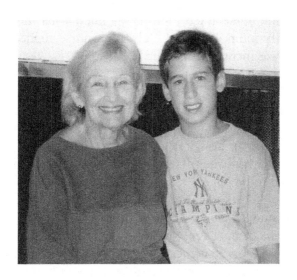

I have heard that Alzheimer's can come and go. Actually it never really disappears, yet there can be moments, even a day, when my mom almost seems not to have any form of dementia. Okay, maybe I am exaggerating a little, although when these moments come it feels like a miracle.

My brother recently told me a cute story about my mom's conversation with a visiting nurse. The nurse was trying to see if my mom needed any other care. My brother and Trudy, her caregiver, were with her when the nurse arrived. She asked my mother many questions, and there were several that Mom could not answer correctly. Then the nurse asked Mom if she knew what month it was. My mom answered "July." The nurse replied that Mom was incorrect, and said it was April.

My feisty mother responded, "If you know what month it is, then why ask me?" As my brother shared this with me, we both laughed. I smiled with pleasure, the pleasure that Mom was still there. She was tough enough to stand up for herself in a cute, innocent way.

Yesterday when I spoke to Mom, her dementia seemed to be gone. I started the conversation by telling her that Logan would be staying at my house for a week while studying for a test. I explained that he had three roommates, and after working all day it was hard for him to study in his apartment. Not only did my mom listen, she also was able to make comments about him and ask me several questions.

Being in the moment, Mom was able to speak about Logan, her one and only grandchild, with pride and deep love. She sentimentally reminisced about how sweet and kind he is. Could this really be a miracle? You see, Mom on most days cannot follow a conversation and even more frequently does not remember her grandson's name.

From far away each day as I speak to her, I try to stimulate her mind by the use of words, questions, and spelling and singing. There are times she rushes me off the phone by saying, "I'm going to hang up now." I answer her that I just called, and Mom says anyway, "I'm going to say goodbye." "That's okay, Mom, just before you hang up, you need to throw me my kisses." And once again that is how our phone calls always end. I catch her kisses, as when I was a young child, and safely place them in my pocket.

I am able to enjoy all the words my mom still can say. I do not question the other parts. What would be the sense? It would only upset me, so I choose to appreciate and savor what I still can call these special moments. Are they miracles? Or perhaps magic? To me it does not really matter.

COMMENTS

Lisa,

Your testimony reached directly to the heart. My mother is also sick Alzheimer's for almost a year. I think the hardest part is seeing the person who previously was strong, intelligent, cheerful become gradually unhappy, confused. This is difficult. But we must help our moms feel safe and surrounded. Make a prayer for them. Thank you, Lisa.

—Alana

I can't read your blogs without tears filling my eyes. My heart and mind drift back to the days we were caring for my mom. But I feel honored to get to share in your journey.

—Holly

Hi Lisa,

You are really lucky. I know what you are talking about. I work as a caregiver in a nursing home in Germany. Some of my clients suffer from dementia, without suffering. They are open-minded, in a good mood, and sometimes able to feel and do things that can change a moment into a miracle. It is just this that makes me go on.

—Paul

Yes, it's truly a disease where we all live in the moments and are grateful for those moments of seeming clarity. Happy Easter!

Wonderful story! Thank you for sharing it with me (and the cyber-world).

—Laurel

Hi Lisa,

My mom suffers from this horrendous disease also, and your story really hit home. So far this has happened to me twice, where she was as lucid as you and I. And like your mom, she no longer knows her grandchildren's names and has been forgetting mine as well. She knows I am her daughter, but that's it. The moments you are speaking of sure seem like miracles to me, and I savor every one of them. Aren't they great? I wish they would last forever. I see her every other day and call her every night to say, "Sweet dreams, I love you." It's not easy.

—Geraldine

April 22, 2012

In Mom's World, Do I Laugh or Cry?

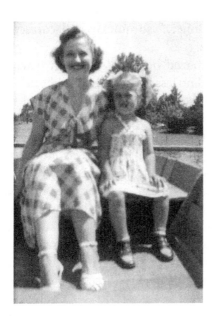

This week in every conversation that I shared with my mom, who has Alzheimer's, I found many joyous and upbeat moments. That is until today.

The week started with my mom and I being excited that I would be coming to see her in twenty-four days. I told her that the countdown began, and she asked me to write it down and send it to her, so she would remember.

There is absolutely no point in doing that, so I decided to start a counting exercise with her every day. "Mom, can you count backwards for me starting at twenty-four and ending at zero?" Mom declared with much enthusiasm, "Of course, I can do that," and she immediately started to count. She started, "Twenty-four, twenty-three, twenty-two, twenty-one…" so quickly and correctly, until she reached zero.

I was amazed how her memory, when it came to counting and no less backwards, just like her spelling, was so refreshingly spontaneous. I then asked her to count backwards skipping two at a time, and she immediately said, "Twenty-four, twenty-two, twenty, eighteen…" until she once again reached zero. I was intrigued and wondered how she was able to do this?

I laughed with her, as I told her that her memory works so well backwards, that maybe she should stand upside down. We then sang some songs, as we both giggled about silly little things we said to each other. Most importantly we shared some wonderful moments. Tomorrow will be twenty-three days until I arrive. I can hardly wait.

The next day I reminded Mom that my brother would be coming to see her. As I continued to joke with her and keep our conversations both simple and light, I told her that she was so lucky to have Gil as her son. Mom answered immediately saying, "Yes, I am one lucky lady, and I love you and Gil so very much." My heart just melted as I said, "We are also so lucky to have you as our mother." She answered with, "Thank you so much for saying that to me." I hung up the phone with a big smile on my face, and a heart filled with much love. Only twenty-two days until I get to see my mom.

The day after when I called, Elaine her caregiver was laughing as she answered the phone. She told me that my mom had just finished telling her all about her own mother. My mom shared how kind, generous, and giving her mom was. All of this was true. As Elaine repeated the conversation to me, my mom chirped in with, "It's true—I would never make up stories."

Elaine handed the phone to Mom. I kidded her about how she was when I was a child. "Oh, you lived near me?" With surprise in my voice, I answered with, "Mom, I lived with you. Who do think you're speaking to?" Mom then said, "I'm not sure."

When I hung up, I turned to my husband and laughed, as I repeated my conversation that I just had with mom. I'm not sure how funny I actually thought it was, although I can get joy from the silly unexpected things that she is still able to say. I guess I'm lucky to still be able to laugh with her or find some joy in her childish ways.

The following day's phone call was a little different. Mom did not know my name. "Mom, I'm your daughter, you actually named me." I heard Trudy, Elaine's daughter, say to her that my name started with the letter L. My mom then said with much question in her voice, "Louise?" (nope) "Lucy?" (nope) "Laura?" (nope), until I said, "My name is Lisa." I then asked, "Mom, what is your son's name?" and Ruthie was able to answer correctly. I then asked her to tell me her first and middle names, and she was able to respond with, "Ruth Esther," which was absolutely correct.

"Okay, Mom, what is my middle name?" She had no idea. I then asked what color hair I had. Mom answered, "Black." I quickly responded that was not my color. Then she said, "Red." Okay, Mom, I've had blond hair for at least the last thirty years. I asked to speak to Trudy, and I said with laughter, "My mom sounded good, yet I guess this is not one of her better days."

As I hung up I felt sadness in my heart. I wondered if I lived closer would she never forget my name. In my heart, I knew the answer. Distance has nothing much to do with what happened today. It's what Alzheimer's does to its victims.

I was able to smile and continue on with my day, although if I say it did not sadden me, I would not be telling the truth. I still keep a smile in my heart, and now have only nineteen more days until I see my mom. I will then be able to give her a big kiss and squeeze her tightly. I do wonder at times if I am the child or the mother. I guess maybe, a little of both.

I get to choose how I handle how I feel. I could laugh or I could cry, or I can cherish all the love that my mom and I still can share, knowing that one day this may no longer be possible. So for today, I'd rather feel the thrill of joy, than the tears of sadness.

COMMENTS

Such an amazingly touching story—amazing that your mom's memory could turn so quickly. The photo of you and your mom is wonderful. Cherish memories. My best to you and your wonderful mom.

—Daniel

I think you sharing your journey with your mother is fantastic and helps so many people realize they aren't alone in their journey, so thank you for sharing.

—Susan

Thank you for sharing your amazing blog! You are a true inspiration!

—Brittney

Lisa,

Hi, I live in Lincolnshire in a village in the United Kingdom. I do read your blogs, and it has helped me a lot. My mum has vascular dementia. She has recently gone to live in a care home as she needed 24/7 care. She is happy she has others to talk to. I have put Mum's bungalow up for sale. It's a five-minute walk away from my home. It is an emotional time. I'm so busy, and I'm a recovering main caregiver. I was helping mum for over five years, unpaid. She had caregivers in. It has left me not right. I'm mentally exhausted. I'm glad I still worked a bit, so hope to get more work ahead. Mum has a great sense of humor. I visit Mum every week and take her surprises, like chocolates, flowers, or I read to her.

—Cynthia

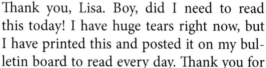

Thank you, Lisa. Boy, did I need to read this today! I have huge tears right now, but I have printed this and posted it on my bulletin board to read every day. Thank you for sharing. I am going to see the positive in all of this, just like you are.

—Suzanne

Does My Mom With Alzheimer's Know It's Mother's Day?

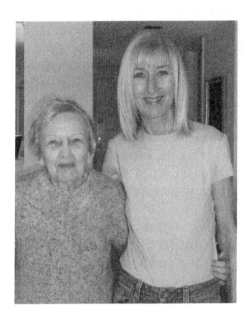

I'll be off to see my mom on Wednesday for Mother's Day. My flight leaves New York early in the morning. As I prepare myself for my trip, I get flashes of all different memories and feelings that are stored up within me. What will Mom be like this time? How much has her Alzheimer's caused her to disappear into her world? Speaking to my mom each day is quite different than living with her. For the most part, my conversations on the phone with my mom are great. Then, of course, there are those other moments. So actually being and living with mom for several days will be quite different. My heart misses her, and my stomach churns both with excitement and nervousness.

This week, my emotions about my mother ran like a river with many inlets. Today's phone call left me feeling exhilarated, yet during the week after she had an episode of incontinence, I fell into an emotion of feeling quite sad and lost. Fortunately she was fine for the rest of the week, as her caregivers realized that they might have overloaded her with too much bran since she had been constipated.

After that episode, I was not able to shake the sadness that I seemed to carry with me for most of the day. I had felt that my mom was no longer whole and had become half a person. How could this be? Where was my mother's journey with Alzheimer's going? What would be happening next? I did not understand, and for the rest of the day, I walked around in a haze, with a lump in my throat and a pain in my heart. Each day when I called, I was frightened, until I was reassured that my mother was doing just fine.

Today, I felt so much joy I wanted to run to a mountain top and spread the words that my mom had just shared with me. She had such a softness and nurturing kindness to her voice. At first we spoke about all the people she could not remember, since most had moved away. Mom said that maybe if she were able to see them, then perhaps she would remember them. "Mom," I declared, "I hope even though I live so far away that you never will forget me." She answered with, "How could I ever forget you?" Then she explained that the most important thing is that we are all well. She continued to say that there was nothing more important than being healthy.

I changed the subject and told her that I would be seeing her in five days as I was coming to celebrate Mother's Day with her. Mom seemed to remember that I had promised to take her for an ice cream sundae. With delight in my voice, and shock that she could remember this, I shouted to her, "Absolutely!" As our phone call was coming to end, Mom then uttered these words: "Do you love me like I love you?" As my heart seemed to break in half, I answered with, "Mom, I love you even more than that." She then started to sing the words as we said our goodbyes.

With much love in my heart, I wanted to take her last words to me and seal them in a bottle for me to open, whenever I so needed to. I knew that after we hung up, Mom would not remember our conversation, nor would she even remember that I will be seeing her in five days. I know that she has no idea that it will soon be Mother's Day. Yet I do, and, for me, my mom will always be that special mother, who for years before she became ill I never even knew I had.

I would like to wish all the moms a very special Mother's Day.

COMMENTS

My mum is also my best friend. She's at an earlier stage than your mum by the sound of it, but I'm having to do more and more for her, such as making her lunch to make sure she eats, etc. When I was picking out a Mother's Day card today, it all of sudden hit me that Mother's Day has become such a hard thing for me. Here I am, a thirty-six-year-old guy standing in the shop welling up, reading cards, thinking about my old mate. It's just not fair for such a great lady to be dealt this. Thank you for sharing your and your beautiful mum's journey. I'll continue to visit this blog even though it's tough. But we have to be tough, don't we, for our mums. You both have a great day.

—Anthony

Thank you for sharing this. This was a different kind of Mother's Day for me too, with Mom so far away with Alzheimer's. Prayers.

—Loren

Thank you for this amazing story. You and your mom have a beautiful bond and love for each other. God bless.

—Nan

Thank you for sharing your amazing blog! You are a true inspiration!

—Shirley

Thank you for lifting my spirits, love. You are a credit to us all. God bless your wonderful mum. I send you both a hug, and please give your mum a cuddle from me too.

—Paulette

Oh Lisa, you don't realize that you are a inspiration to us. You definitely touched my heart!

—Walter

Thank you for sharing your amazing blog! You are a true inspiration!

—Beryl

Hi, just wanted to say I read your blog regularly. I looked after my uncle for twelve years. He had macular degeneration and for the last five had Alzheimer's. Sadly, he died in May, aged eighty-six. We always joked about him getting a telegram from the Queen when he was a hundred years old, a custom we have in Britain when one reaches that age. But the uncle I knew had left years before. Your mum seems such a lovely person, and I wish things could have been different for her and for you. All I can say is treasure every day. I found with my uncle there was always something he did or said that made me smile. Anyway, take care.

—Angela

Your mother, her wise replies, her not recalling your calls or visits, and your gratitude for her and the deep love you share, all remind me of my past journey that ended in 2010. I feel so much love for my beautiful mom and know I missed too much. I was there every day except for a few vacation breaks, but I sure wish I had found a place for us both, so she could have woken up and gone to bed knowing she had me by her side. I do feel guilt over having her in a care-home. In the initial stages she was feisty, fearful, and wouldn't allow me to give her the help she needed. After she became severely sick (bladder infection caused sepsis) and in ICU, I placed her in a home. Nevertheless, I know I had love, advocacy, and care for her on a daily basis. After she passed, my distant and nonexistent sister (wouldn't even call) came in to undermine my whole journey. She also hired an attorney, made false accusations I couldn't disprove, and got the majority of funds left. The case took the last two years; I really have just now fully began missing my mama, and reading your blog brings me beautiful memories of her. The end had so much suffering (she had a fall and there were complications). I did move her in my home and slept by her side. So keep writing your blog. It helps me recall the simple and sweet, truthful replies of my mama and her heart of gold. Mothers are so precious!

—Anne

The Distance Between Us

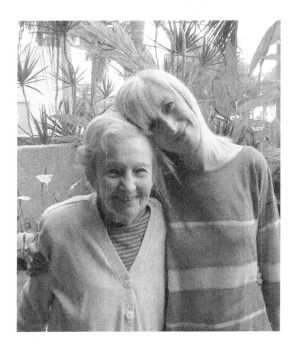

It's amazing to me that three days before my visit to see my mom, she asked me each time that I called when would I be coming to visit. I knew in my heart that embedded somewhere in her memory she knew that I was coming to see her. Mom and I for the last two weeks had been counting backwards till I would be arriving at her home. She sounded vibrant and filled with much life and excitement. Even if I were imagining all of this, it did not matter, for I could feel in my heart and soul the same joy as I waited for my plane to take off.

My visit to her house several days before Mother's Day left me with different emotions. While I was with her, I felt much love, mixed with some pain and frustration. On a very upbeat note, my mom was doing wonderfully. At moments when she refused to brush her teeth or get dressed, I had to remind myself that her yelling at me that she was not a child was frustrating to both of us. I laughed, I cried, and the love I felt towards her touched me deeply.

I witnessed her as she danced and shared the same story over and over again with my dear friend Alana, who came to visit us. Mom was especially vibrant. Alana described her as "both beautiful and spunky," this being the first time they ever met.

The following morning when Mom awoke, I was lying on the floor while I did my daily exercises. The day before Mom assisted me as I had her count to one hundred while I performed my Pilates moves. With much enthusiasm that morning, Mom was so excited to see me. She immediately joined in and started to count to one hundred. As I lay on the towel, she spoke these words: "Seeing your face and having you here are both very comforting to me." I melted from her sentimental words.

As I stood up to continue my routine, she then asked, "Who is your mother?" With amazement I looked at her and said, "Mom, you are my mother, and I love you deeply." Mom replied, "I love you also." I then asked her my name. After her calling me Lisa for two days, at least a thousand times she said, "It's on the tip of my tongue, although at this second I cannot remember it." "Mom," I said, "my name is Lisa."

After my return to New York, I shared with my husband that my mom was filled with moments where she was so lucid, and then there were the other moments that seemed to come and go. Yet I felt quite grateful on how well she seemed to be doing. I guess I got lucky this trip, because there have been other visits when my mom's Alzheimer's seemed to take control.

The next morning she sounded so excited to hear from me. I shared that I missed her counting for me as I exercised. Mom replied, "It's funny how you get used to doing something." "I guess so, Mom, although I really do miss you." As our phone call came to an end, she did once again ask, "When will I see you?" I thought to myself that I had just left, yet I answer with, "I'll see you in a couple of weeks." Mom then uttered the words, "That's great, because you know that I love seeing you."

As of this moment, it is not the fact that my mom has Alzheimer's that upsets me, it's that I live so far away and do not have the opportunity to go and see her each day. Could it be that I miss her so much because today is Mother's Day? No, I know the answer to that. It is the fact that whatever day or time, the distance between us still remains the same.

COMMENTS

Thanks for sharing your story. It's heart-warming to read of your love and compassion. The ability to appreciate the moment is a gift and to not get totally frustrated at times is a blessing. From an early onset Lewy body dementia patient.

—Anonymous

You expressed the frustrations of Alzheimer's so beautifully in your conclusion. It's true. No matter how close or far away you are to your dear loved one, there will always be that distance. My best to you as you cope with this devastating illness.

—Bethany

What an awesome story! Agreed that the sentiment was shared beautifully. We wish you love, patience, and hope. Thank you so much for sharing such an honest and heart-warming story.

—Maureen

Lisa,

Thank you so much for sharing your journey, I found out about your blog just now, and it offers the hope and courage my family and

I need at present. My grandmother will be moving into a nursing home this week. My mom and I (her caregiver) found out today that a room has just become available. It is logically the right decision and it's been discussed for a while, but it still feels devastating. She's been with us ever since I can remember. Reading your stories gives me so much hope. Thank you again, with much love and gratitude.

—Margaret

So Sweet and Tender

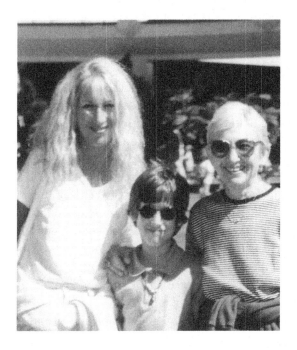

Since my last visit my mom has been asking me almost every day when I will be coming to see her. The truth is that I will not be returning for at least three to four months. Yet I do not share these thoughts with her. This time when she asked, my answer was within a few weeks. She replied, "What does a few weeks mean?" I quickly answered her by saying I would be visiting in four weeks, although I knew this was not true. She then whispered so sweet and tender, "That's good, for four weeks is pretty soon." Ruthie did like my answer, and I had no fear that she could remember and hold me to this time frame.

Of course there is some sadness that I did not tell her the truth, and even more that we live so far away from one another. How special it would be if I could see her at least once a week as my brother is able to do.

My mom said that she remembered that I was at her home, yet she could not say when or for how many days I visited. I knew from her caregivers that for the first week after I left, she walked around calling my name and looking for me.

We continued our phone call, and I had Ruthie spelling from A–Z using countries, cities, and states. I started off with Arizona, then Barcelona, Connecticut, and onward. When I asked her to spell New York, she started to sing the lyrics to "New York, New York," and when I reached San Francisco, she sang, "I Left My Heart in San Francisco." These songs have become familiar to most of us, like national anthems.

When Mom did not understand my pronunciation of some words that I asked her to spell, she sharply told me to speak English. She made me laugh, and I did feel joyous for she sounded so aware and alert. She was into our spelling game and scored a ninety-five—for her, almost perfection.

If my mom did not have Alzheimer's and she said what she said to me, I might have felt annoyed. Now it is quite different. As far as I am concerned, my mom can do no wrong. I just appreciate and cherish every word that comes from her lips.

On this particular day, she was as sharp as a tack and filled with much clarity. I once again wondered if it was all the coconut oil that my brother has her caregivers give her each day. He read an article about how it had helped someone with Alzheimer's. So he immediately bought it for her. At this point I do not mind the things he tries, certainly since something might work. No one really knows.

I ended our phone call with telling her how much I loved her and said, "Mom, I wish that I lived close to you." Ruthie answered, "Me too. Who knows, maybe one day we will." With a smile and a wish, I whispered back to her, "Mom, wouldn't that really be nice?"

Her sweetness and tenderness have me miss her so. My mom's strength and courage has inspired me. She has become my hero. My love and appreciation for who she is just amazes me. Alzheimer's may have stolen her memory, yet Alzheimer's cannot steal the enormous love I feel for her.

I am so fortunate to also feel all the love she has for me, and I am sure that she still can remember how very much I love her. Tomorrow when I awake, although I will not be able to see her, I will still be able to pick up my phone and hear her sweet and tender words. For this I am quite grateful.

COMMENTS

I can't help but to think that Alzheimer's, in some ways, brings people back to almost a childlike state of mind, when at times you can't tell them the truth since they simply wouldn't understand the truth or accept it—which is okay. I have seen some similarities with how you treat someone with a memory disorder and how you would treat a young child. This is not to say at all that there is a loss of preciousness or sweetness as we advance in age and possibly develop these awful disorders, but unfortunately, we probably have to change how we act and react around mom and dad when it happens. I am so glad, though, that you seem to apparently have good days with her still, and that she is still communicating. You so obviously love her tremendously.

—Danny

Thank you for your story. I sometimes wonder, what would happen if I were to take my mom to East Germany, where she was born and now is asking for all the time. In September last year, we talk her to the seaside of The Netherlands. She liked the ocean and the wind. Suddenly she had a twinkle in her eyes. She liked it and also to see the children playing in the sand. We went there only for a day, and we will never forget how happy she was for a moment. One day later, she didn't know anymore that we went away for a ride to the seaside. The journey to East Germany, where she was born, is long, and I am not sure whether she can bear it. I have been thinking about for few weeks, and I don't know how to decide. But I could imagine that it would be better for all to be in here and now situations. It's great to read how deep your love for your mom is. Thank you. I wish you all the best. May God bless you all.

—Marnie

Wonderful story. I so relate to what you are feeling.

—Shari

Lisa,

I love your writing style and can relate to so much of what you say. My mother has had Alzheimer's for about the past eight years. As you said, it's hard to tell exactly when it took hold. There were signs galore, but I wanted so badly to believe it was just "normal aging" (despite the fact that she was only sixty-eight years old). In any case, I'm going to post a link to your blog on my own blog. After reading just a few posts, I feel like we have so much in common. Thank you for sharing your personal experiences; I'll be visiting often. I'm sure that you are bringing comfort to many going through the same thing.

—Linette

This is so touching. It made me cry.

—Barbara

I've been a fan of your blog for quite a while. I love your honesty and find it incredibly touching that you are sharing such an intimate journey. I'm sure it has helped many many people view their journeys with Alzheimer's and their loved ones very differently and had as incredible effect for them. Thank you so much.

—Sherri Ann

She Really Makes Me Smile

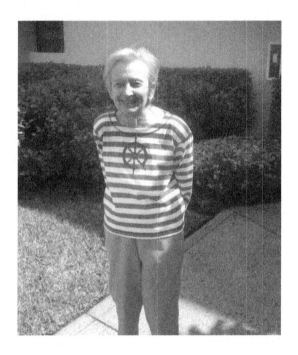

"Hi Mom, how are you?" "Lisa, is that you?" "Yes, Mom, it's your beautiful daughter calling her favorite mom to see how you are doing." "Lisa, when are you coming to see me?" "Mom," I fibbed, "I'll be coming in four weeks." Mom replied, "That's great because I really miss you."

I feel a pang in my heart because I know that I will

not be returning to see my mom for several months. I can get away with this white lie, because Ruthie has no recollection of what I just said, let alone when I lasted visited . Actually my mom cannot remember anything anymore. "Mom, I live too far away, and I was just at your home six weeks ago." "I really do not remember," she answers. "It feels like a very long time ago."

"Well, Mom, you do have a special person coming to visit you today." "Who?" "Your son Gil is coming to visit with his girlfriend." Mom breaks in with, "Gil has a girlfriend?" "Yes, Mom, and we both met her when I visited six weeks ago." "What is his girlfriend's name?" "Her name is Rochelle, and she's very nice." I mention to her that they will be coming with their two dogs. "Why?" "Because the dogs want to visit you also. Please be careful that you do not step on them." We both find this quite amusing, and start to giggle.

"Mom, would you like to come and visit me in New York?" "No, not now," she replies, as she goes on to describe how she once lived there many years ago. She remembers looking out the window and watching as things went by. "Well, Mom, I remember you and I going to the museums, the theater, the top of the Empire State Building, and taking the buses and subways all over the city." "Lisa, I did that? I do not remember, for it was so long ago." "I do, Mom, and I also remember how much you enjoyed yourself."

Unfortunately if she did any of these things today, she still would not remember. This is what Alzheimer's has done to her. Her mind once filled with beautiful visions has now become a blank canvas. A lifetime of her memories that have all been washed away disappeared as if they never did exist.

"Mom, I love you. I'll speak to you later." "Okey dokey," she says and answers with, "I love you even more."

I have just approached the Alzheimer's Association offices in the city. I am here for a meeting to get involved with a project to help spread awareness with them, for September is Alzheimer's Month. We want to paint the town purple and to spread our word for all to hear.

It's strange how I hung up with my mom the very moment that I approached the entrance to their offices. As I entered, I had plastered across my face a huge smile and a heart filled with much warmth. I realized how almost every day when I speak to her, we share these silly, touching, and funny conversations. Our conversations make little sense, yet they seem to lighten our hearts and make us laugh. We share a laugh from within that leaves our hearts filled with much pleasure and joy.

My mom probably forgets immediately what we just shared, yet for me I walk away feeling enlightened and carefree. When my mom was free of this disease, these lighthearted, fun conversations did not exist. I was too busy wanting to get off the phone, and now every time that I speak to her I hang up with feelings of so much love and happiness.

As strange as it sounds, there for me is much joy in whatever time we still have together, for this special lady can really make me smile.

COMMENTS

What a wonderful tribute to your mom. God bless you.

—Lana

I loved your story about your mother and you. keep up the good work.

—Ellie

Love every single post of your blog. Keep up the good job.

—PositiveMed

My Man, I Loved Him So

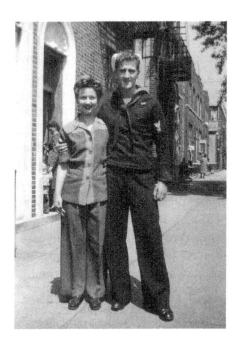

Today when I spoke to my mom, I mentioned that it was my birthday in eight days. When I questioned her about what day I was born and how old I would be, Mom said that she had no recollection of any of it. I whispered to her my age, and with humor, she answered, "You're catching up to me." I giggled at her quick and witty response.

When I phoned, she and her caregiver Elaine had just been watching a love story on the television. Elaine was so excited to share with me what my mom had just finished saying. Mom said to her that the movie was a beautiful love story. She continued to tell her that she lost her husband a long time ago (seventeen years to be exact) and that she really missed him. The next thing she said was that she'd do anything to have him back.

What my ears had just heard sent chills up and down my spine. Out of my sometimes fear to not cause her any unnecessary pain, I avoid bringing up my dad to her. At times when I have, my mom usually says that she cannot remember him. No matter how many times I have heard this from her, to be married for almost fifty years and to have shared a family and lifetime together and still not be able to remember it still amazes me.

The saving grace for me, and of course for her, is that I know deep in my heart that whatever memories she had of my dad are now long forgotten. She can no longer feel her broken heart or any unnecessary pain.

"Hi, Mom, I heard you just watched a movie that you really enjoyed." Mom answered with, "Yes, it was very good." "What was it about?" I inquired. I then heard my mom ask Elaine to please tell me what the movie was about, for she could not remember.

The feelings of her remembering my dad were all but washed away, almost like a passing rain shower or, even more, like a rainbow that quickly fades away.

Mom and Dad were married in 1942, when she had just turned eighteen years old. My dad was turning twenty-one and soon to be shipping off with the Navy. They were married for a little shy of fifty years, and now for Mom it seems to be a life that has been taken away. I wonder how such a disease can destroy a lifetime of memories.

Hopefully one day researchers in the medical field will be able to find a cure, so others will be able to hold on to the memories of their lives and all their loved ones. So Dad, if Mom could remember her most recent words, I'm sure she would say again, "My man, I loved him so."

COMMENTS

What a nice story, Lisa. At least you now know that she does remember your father—maybe she just needs something like that movie to nudge it from her memory bank. Your stories are so inspiring. Keep them coming!

—Kathleen

What a sweet mom you have. I love how she smiles in some of the pictures. It brings joy to my heart to see her smile despite this awful disease.

—Ginger

Lisa,

You and your mom are doing a wonderful job. Your story has gone around the world via Facebook. It is inspirational! Thanks so much for sharing.

All the best,
Holly

≈≈≈

Dear Lisa,

I saw the post you wrote about your mom on a Facebook page. It was beautiful and moving. I am an eldercare placement specialist in Los Angeles for sixteen years specializing in dementia and Alzheimer's residents. Your mom sounds like a peach. Additionally, my dad has Alzheimer's, so I relate to your blog both personally and professionally. Thanking you for sharing your journey.

—Steffanie

I Feel Mom Drifting Away

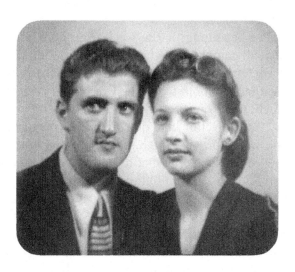

My mom will be eighty-eight years old in fourteen days. For this I am quite grateful. Yet for the last few weeks, I have felt how she is starting to drift further away. One could say she's like a boat lost at sea or caught in the midst of a dense fog.

Yes, we still have our special moments, and I can still hear the sound of joy and laughter coming from her as we speak. I just notice that they are becoming less frequent. At times her voice sounds more lethargic and somewhat listless. Perhaps it is that she is moving further along with her Alzheimer's, and also being eighty-eight makes her no spring chicken.

In the beginning of the week, my mom sounded disoriented, complaining about back pains. She did not know where she lived and only wanted to go back home, for fear that her mom would be worried about her. We were fortunate to realize that Mom was having another urinary tract infection, and quickly got her on an antibiotic. We went down this path several months ago, so we are now educated about what to do for her. It is several days later now, and Mom sounds "back to normal."

Mom will sometimes kid around with me and tell me that I am catching up to her in age. "How about your height?" I ask of her. Mom, who is less than five feet tall, responds with, "Who knows? Maybe I still will grow." At moments like that, her humor warms my heart.

I try my best to keep her mind stimulated. Mom has been an excellent speller and always had a great vocabulary. She seems to still get ninety percent of the words she spells correct. Yet when I ask her to spell Portugal, she says to me, "What's that? I never heard of it." Or she'll say, "What is a lobster?" which mom use to love to eat. "Mom, can you spell 'illusion'?" "I never heard of that word." "Okay, Mom, spell 'delusion,'" which she was able to do as simple as one, two, three.

Her voice seems more tired, and there are more days when she wants to take quite few a naps. Mom was someone who never napped. I wonder if she is up all hours of the night, since I'm aware that people with Alzheimer's have awkward sleeping patterns. Day is night and nights can be day. They do not realize the difference, as if the times of day are all rolled into one.

On the other side of this cloud is still some sunshine. Mom asked when I am coming to visit, after I had just described how foggy it was outside. She then was able to respond that I shouldn't come until the sky brightens, because she would never want anything to happen to me.

"Mom, you can really break my heart, when you say things like that." I continued with, "Do you know how very much I love you?" She answered with, "No, I know you love me, but I do not understand what 'much' means." I try to explain with a little surprise in my voice. I quickly move past this conversation.

No matter which way our conversations go, and no matter how much she is drifting away, I still hold on to how lucky I am. On most days, we are still able to speak and laugh. I cherish all our silly conversations and delight in the moments of joy that we still can share. I have no idea how long my mom will be able to remember who I am or my name, so today as always I am thankful for all that we still can share as she seems to drift away.

COMMENTS

> Hi, my name is Joanne, and I live in Canada. I found your blog recently, and I feel a connection with you. My mom has Alzheimer's, has been diagnosed for six years, and is only

seventy-seven. She is in a nursing home an hour from me. I am finding it so hard, and I know that you understand. Thanks for sharing your heart, your emotions, and your humor. I am going to visit my mom today. I cherish every visit and hope against hope that she knows me today.

—Joan

A very touching post.

—Cara

Thank you for your positive comments. I too need to focus on the good things each day- and cherish the memories. Congratulations on your efforts to maintain normality

—Auggie

Just found your blog through the Walk to End Alzheimer's Facebook page, and I cried as I read this today. My mom passed away seven years ago yesterday, after eight years with early onset Alzheimer's. Your stories of times with your dear mom touch my heart in a way I can't explain. You will be in my prayers as you continue this journey with your sweet mom.

—Henrietta

I am really lucky that so far this has not affected our family. My grandparents are now both ninety, and I have to say there are little flickers that my grandad is starting to forget things more and more. However, who wouldn't at ninety? Really heart-wrenching insight into living with this cruel illness.

—Anonymous

Great heart-wrenching read. My nan has had Alzheimer's for at least ten years now, and it's pretty tough to watch them drift further away while being totally powerless to do anything. But you have to try and take it your stride. Birthdays can be tough on her, as she's not sure what's happening (plus refuses to be told she's ninety), and there's a fair few people about, but you'll get the odd time when her face lights up and she's remembered/clicked with something. That makes it all worthwhile.

—Anonymous

Glimmers of a Rainbow

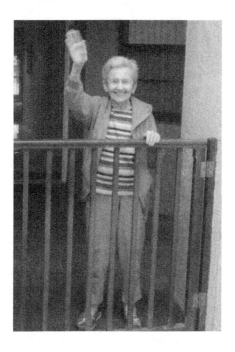

Sometimes when dark clouds start to clear, the sky opens up to glimmers of a rainbow. This is how my mom's week ended, after the antibiotic she has been on started to work. Mom appeared listless in the beginning of the week, only wanting to sleep her days away. That was before we were aware that she had a urinary tract infection.

Not anymore. The sounds of her laughter and joy could certainly fill the size of a ballroom. Mom was reciting to me a rhyme that she recently made up. "Mister, mister, where did you meet your sister?" She repeated it over and over again, with much expression and humor in her voice. Each time that she sang her new rhyme—"Mister, Mister, where did you meet your sister?"—we would both giggle, as she rejoiced with her newfound verses. Even her caregiver Trudy was laughing hysterically.

Just hearing the sound of her joy and happiness delighted me, sending thrills up and down my spine. She sounded so alive, as if she were having an adrenaline rush or maybe about to run a marathon race. Either way the excitement that she showed brought a needed smile to my face and lightness to my heart. The prior week, I knew that my mom was having a rather hard time.

Alzheimer's is such a strange disease and one that I do not truly understand. One day my mom can be lethargic, and the next day she can be dancing the night away. I never know how long these moments of aliveness can last. Nor do I want to know. I just try to go with the flow of Mom's ups and downs.

I wish that every day would be an up day for her. This I know is not possible. I find it hard to even imagine how in some ways she is so alive, yet in other ways there is not much that exists in her life.

Mom will be eighty-eight years old at the end of this week. Except for having Alzheimer's and macular degeneration, she is in rather good health. She never seems to complain about anything, and on her good days there is always joy and laughter that resonates from her being. The only thing that she will say to me is that she cannot remember much of anything.

Actually mom remembers very little of anything. For me the most important thing is that she still remembers me. I know that this is a gift to be cherished, a gift that may one day be taken away. Yet today I choose to remain happy. It's almost like when I see the glimmers of rainbows forming in the sky. I see all the beauty and do not remember the storm that just passed by.

COMMENTS

Lisa,

I was one of those daughters who came to that point when my mom did not know who I was and would inquire, "Where is Serena?" Even twenty-five years later, it still causes a tear to fall and a heart to ache, but I knew her. She was very young, sixty-six when she passed. Dad had gone on the year before at sixty. They married not ever inquiring as to the age of either of them and only meeting once before the ceremony. Theirs was a war romance of letters and poetry during WWII. But they lived, loved, and enjoyed life and each other. My brother also passed at sixty-one, so I and my husband and two children and grandchildren go on and remember the times when they were here with us and the smiles and love they gave. It will get better as time heals. Advice is cheap, but the one thing I can say is love each moment and make it precious to both of you. You will thank yourself for that someday. My heart goes out to you, along with my prayers.

—Serena

Lisa,

Thank you for sharing your world. My heart goes out to you and I think it wonderful the amount of people you touch by sharing so unselfishly all that you feel and experience.

—Linda

Thanks for sharing, Lisa. For folks like us, every day is Alzheimer's Day. Keep the posts coming. Your stories are amazing, and you are helping spread awareness. Thank you.

—Homewatch CareGivers Columbus

Life Is Short—Be Happy

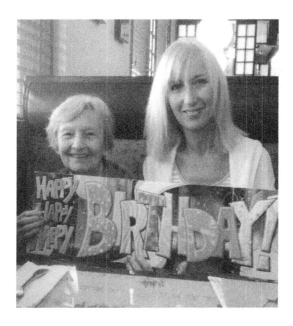

The picture above is from a birthday we celebrated together two years ago, while I was visiting my mom in Florida. Today she turned eighty-eight years young. This year I remained in New York during her birthday (which was yesterday). The best I could do was send her a special birthday card filled with much love and affection and to sing her the "Happy Birthday" song. As we approached her birthday, it was in many ways quite different.

The week started when my mom's caregiver Trudy called around 8:30 a.m. to tell me that she phoned for an ambulance to take Mom to the hospital. She had cleared the decision with my brother Gil.

When she arrived, she found Ruthie to be a little disoriented and complaining terribly about pain in her neck. Trudy discovered that my mom had several bruises and black and blue marks on her arms, wrists, and fingers. We all wondered what had happened to her, and since she could not tell us, we all assumed that Mom must have fallen down.

The medics arrived, and Ruthie was at least able to tell them her birth date and her name as they strapped her to a stretcher and placed her in the ambulance. Several hours later when I spoke to the emergency room doctor, they were discharging Mom and sending her home. The doctor said that they ran many tests, with X-rays, an MRI, urine, and blood, and he was pleased to say that everything was normal. Yes, in the doctor's world, "normal," and in ours, "except for having Alzheimer's." Thankfully, nothing appeared to be broken.

I spoke to everyone several times that day from the hospital and later when Mom was back at home. The next two days she appeared to be so weak that she had trouble walking to the bathroom. We had her caregivers, who normally stay for twelve hours, sleep over with her for several days. By day three, Mom was starting to bounce back. She was walking much better and started laughing and singing along with me as we practiced her birthday song.

What struck me the most with this week was the several comments my mom had made about life and being alive. The day she came back home from the hospital, she was rambling on about things that made absolutely no sense. When I mentioned that she was in the hospital, she said, "No, I was never in the hospital." I thought that all the strange things she was describing were in some way related to the nurses, the X-ray machines, the fear of being in an ambulance, things that she was not able to express. Yet as clear as day, my mom, in between speed-talking, said to me, "Life is short, so you just need to remember to be happy." I hung up the phone, turned to my husband with amazement, and thought how profound it was what my mom had just said.

The next day, somewhere in our conversation, Mom said to me that she wanted to be alive. With lightness in my voice, I told her that she was very alive, for to whom else was I speaking? Finally on the day before her birthday, as we practiced singing her birthday song. As we got to the end of, "How old are you now, how old are you now?" Mom answered with, "Old enough to be alive, and thank God."

All these phrases she kept saying about life and living only left me to wonder what she had felt was happening to her this week. These are feelings that she can no longer share or express for they just disappear from her memory. All the things she described to me, I truly believe for her, were a statement of wanting to live. Mom was not ready to die.

So, Mom, I toast you on your birthday. As you just recently said to me, I will remember that "life is short, so we need to be happy." Yes, my sweet, loving mom, once again your words become wisdom to my ears. I just want to wish you a very Happy Birthday, and to let you know how very much I love and cherish you. I do not know how many more we will be able to celebrate together, yet for number eighty-eight, it stays in my heart as a very special one.

COMMENTS

Happy birthday to your mom, Lisa. This blog is special. The love you show is special, and it made my day.

—Joyce

This post brought tears to my eyes. I'm the caregiver of a terminally ill parent. Thank God, she is still very much alert and mentally active, although confusion is one of the major symptoms of her disease (multiple myeloma). As many of her other faculties diminish (more quickly as of late), I find myself sometimes startled by the emotional intensity of some of our exchanges—always loving and honest. My mother has always been the strength and heart of our family, so I feel I owe her all the care and consideration I can muster. I was struck by the strong resonance I felt in your words. It is hard to put into words, but I truly feel I have learned more about life, love, and the human condition in these last few months than in all the years that have proceeded them. Feeling the depth and earnestness of love in the eyes of a dying parent has a way of burning away a lot of the dross and getting to what is important. Like you, I can attest that my mom is my hero. Thank you so much for sharing your experience.

—Rolan

Lisa,

I've been following your blog for some time now. To be honest, some days I can't bear to click on the link. I don't feel strong enough to read what are, more times than not, words of loving amazement, understanding, and acceptance of all that your beautiful mom is/ has become. Some days I feel too upset, too distraught, too guilt-ridden, or too much in denial perhaps. I don't know. But I want you to know that since I first came across your blog, at a time when I was in a much darker place than I am this year, I have learned so much from your experiences and from your expression of honest emotion. Thank you so much. I cannot write about my own mom's descent into Alzheimer's as you've done. I might do that someday I hope. But I have begun to turn a corner in my grief for the mom I once was so close to, the mom I still love but who is quite lost to me. I'm learning to treasure what we still have. It's tough. But your posts show me that I have much left to learn from the woman who has always been my greatest ally. Please know that your posts are making a difference, I am sure of it, to any and all who come across it here in cyberspace. God bless.

—Julie

Because I Love You

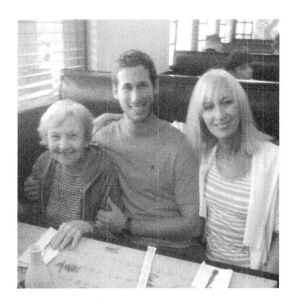

My mom's greeting to me directly after saying our good morning hellos was, "When are you coming to see me?" "Mom," I fibbed as usual, "in a couple of weeks." "That's wonderful, and who are you coming with?" "My husband," I replied. "You're married?" "Yes, Mom, I've been married for thirty years." "I can't believe you're married, you look so young. You look like a baby."

As I smiled to myself and felt all the sentimental love coming my mom, I also flashed on when I was a little girl, which was many years ago. I thought of my mom in her youth and all the things we did together. That was then and this is now.

She then asked where I lived, and I answered, "New York." Mom was able to have a moment of memory for she answered, "I used to come to visit you a lot in New York." *That's true, Mom*, I thought, *and you also were born and raised here. New York was your home.*

Mom lived here till she was sixty-two years old. She moved right before I became pregnant with her one and only grandchild. Logan is his name, named after her dad Louis. He will be turning twenty-five in several months. Today, with all the love she has felt for him and all the special moments they shared, he is just a fading memory in her life.

Last week when I mentioned Logan's name, she said it sounded familiar to her. Her grandson that she so adored is now just a glimpse of a shadow in her world. I know in my heart that all her love is still there for him, it's just that she cannot connect all the pieces. Sometimes when we speak of her grandchild, she thinks that he is still a young child. She will ask why I allow him to do some of the things I share with her. She cannot believe how old he is, what he looks like, or his stature of being six feet tall.

Deciding to lighten the conversation and to have some fun, I asked Ruthie if she'd like to live with me in New York. Mom used to express that her wishes were to remain in Florida. This time to my surprise, she said, "How would I get there?" "Well, Mom, I could come and get you." "When would that be?" she questioned. "Maybe soon." "Okay, let me think about it." Of course this conversation, like so many others, quickly faded into the distance. The next time we spoke, Mom had no memory of it.

Alzheimer's, now that I can see what it has stolen from her life and her existence, still leaves me with the question of, "How can this disease just eat away your life, as if it never existed?" It is mind boggling to me.

As our phone call came to an end, Mom softly whispered to me, "Please come visit. I have a home you can stay in. Lisa, you know that you can come whenever you want, because I love you."

At that moment this little lady, who is no longer five feet tall, broke my heart. I wanted to pick her up and hold her in my arms and tell her that everything will be okay. Yes, I know that is not the way this illness usually ends. Yet for now, I still can hear Mom speak those tender words to me. For me, at the moment, this is all I need. I feel all her love and deeply cherish all that we still have, no matter how little it may be.

COMMENTS

This is absolutely touching.

—Anonymous

My ma has dementia. I am her caregiver as well as being her daughter. She is a couple of years into it and at the moment still remembers who we all are. She has difficulty getting words out that she wants to say or forgets what she wants to say. It is getting more and more like a game of charades. I love her so much, and it scares me what I have yet to face. But I am enjoying every day whilst she does still remember me and will let me help. My heart goes out to you.

—Alicia

What Becomes
of the Broken Hearted?

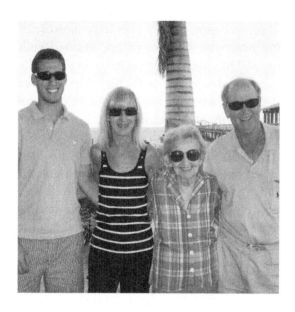

This picture was taken in October 2011, with my son Logan, me, Mom, and my brother Gil. Mom looks happy. What I remember about this day was that she did not want to leave her home. We had to force it upon her. Although she's smiling in the picture, I would not say that she was really thrilled to be out. I think she enjoyed being with all of us, yet having lunch by the ocean and feeling the warm breezes blow by meant nothing to her. For me,

I loved the day, because it is not that often that the four of us can get together, especially since we live in different states.

In the beginning of this week I phoned my mother because I wanted to share something exciting with her. Logan had just gotten an apartment with his girlfriend. I was feeling so happy, yet my eyes were moist with tears. My little boy, who has grown up, finished college, is working, and has been living on his own for the last four years, was now taking his next "big" step. As I see it, he and Julia, after dating for two years, were now making a deeper commitment to one another.

As Logan has taken each step in his life, they are both exciting and thrilling to me and are quite sentimental. I called my mom to share all this excitement with her. With much enthusiasm, I shared everything, including my happiness as well as my heart pangs. I know that since she is a mother, she had to have similar feelings when my brother and I took each new step.

While speaking to her, the phone just went silent. Mom said nothing. She didn't even make a comment, which she has been able to do, nor did she give any words of wisdom. There was just dead silence. Mom had put the phone down. Her caregiver picked up the phone and put her back on. I once again in a more simplified matter shared everything with her. I then asked if she had anything to say. Wasn't she listening? Didn't she care? Couldn't I speak to Mom and have her be excited with me?

Not this time, and probably not too many times in the future. I questioned why couldn't she be there for me? I used to love to call her when I needed advice or had something exciting to tell her. Those days seem to be long gone. I felt both sad and lost, and I felt like crying. I only wanted my mom back. Is that too much to ask? The answer is yes. Alzheimer's seems to destroy inch by inch someone's entire being.

My thoughts went deep and dark, and I was beginning to feel such anger to this disease. I had to pull myself together and get back to the lighter side of life, or I could drive myself crazy. Yes, I had to remember other moments that Mom and I can share. I quickly thought of the laughter and all the words we say to one another that are filled with deep love.

Maybe this was just a bad day for her. Tomorrow will be better. I must lighten up and stay on the brighter side. I wish that I could remove this horrific disease from my mom's being, yet I know that's impossible.

September is World Alzheimer's Month. We all to need to help spread awareness around the world, and find a cure for Alzheimer's. Hopefully this will happen in my lifetime, and if not, certainly for future generations.

I'd like to send to all the families who have a loved one with this disease, and to all their caregivers, much love. Although I felt a broken heart for my mom, I know deep in my heart, that broken hearts can heal.

COMMENTS

Wonderful story. I so relate to what you are feeling.

—Lisa

⸻

I have been planning to call home, to talk to Mom and Dad for almost two weeks now. The calls are tough, but shame on me for not making them more often as you do. I admire that about you. You keep calling. It's too late now, but I promise I will call my folks tomorrow.

—Anna

⸻

Your blog and your story is an inspiration.
—The Alzheimer Society of Manitoba

⸻

Hi—I just read some of your thoughts about your mom. It helps to read about other people's relationships. I see so many similarities—at times, I wonder, am I imagining things or over re-acting to something. My husband can seem so normal for moments and then be so different. I wonder, did I make a wrong decision when I placed him in a Memory Care Unit, and then I remember all the reasons why I did. At other times, I think, maybe I could take him home and hire help to take care of him. And then I just feel guilty. I feel so alone without him here. I have family and friends, but it is not the same.

I thought I would feel relief and I think my family expect me to feel relief but I feel like a piece of me is gone.
Thank you for sharing your feelings. It helps.
—Louanne

Hello,

You don't know me, but I saw your blog that you posted on the San Diego Alzheimer's Association page. I read through some of your blog postings and love that you are documenting your time with your mum. I've been around people suffering from various types of dementia including those with Alzheimer's my whole life. My mum has cared for them for over thirty years. I did volunteer work with them throughout my childhood and teenage years. More recently I worked as a caregiver for a woman with Alzheimer's for two years. It was the hardest but most rewarding job I've had, she was family to me—like a grandmother, I loved her to pieces and vice versa. Sadly she passed away in spring of last year, shortly before her ninetieth birthday. I've been working as a volunteer and intern with the Alzheimer's Association since July of this year and love it. It is such a wonderful organization, and everyone I've worked with has been super nice. I hope to work with them full time after I finish with school. Anyway, I just wanted to send a wee message/hello after reading your blog. Have a lovely week!

—Suzi

Interviewing My Mom
With Alzheimer's

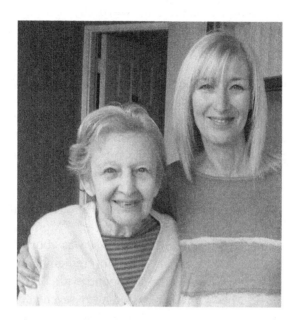

"Mom, what does it feel like not to be able to remember something?" She answered, "It is not always so bad not to remember everything." *Wow*, I thought. Several years before I had presented a similar question to her, for I often wondered what it must be like. I too sometimes forget some simple things, and for a second I think, *Do I also have the beginnings of dementia?*

I quickly joke about it, although deep inside the question still remains.

I have no fear of asking her any questions, for I know that it will not upset her. Immediately after I ask her something, it disappears from her memory. Her answer to this same question several years ago was quite touching. Mom had said, "I know that whatever happened yesterday to me had to be nice, whether I can remember it or not."

Back to the present, I continue with, "Mom, does any of this frighten you?" Her quick reply is, "No, it's not scary because if you cannot remember something, you just don't remember it." With such wisdom, Mom was able to answer me so easily. She then started to reminisce about her own mother and growing up in Williamsburg and Coney Island, which are both located in Brooklyn, New York.

"Mom, do you remember your mother's name?" "Of course, it was Pauline Schnitzer." "Mom, what's your name?" "Ruth Schnitzer." "What was your father's name?" She simply says, "I cannot remember." With much surprise in my voice, I respond with, "His name was Louis." My own father passed away seventeen years ago, yet I wonder if she even knows his name. She must, for it's my dad, and they were married for almost fifty years. I became brave and questioned her, yet she does not remember.

"Mom, how many brothers or sisters do you have?" "I have both a brother and a sister." Wrong again. My mom had only one (younger) brother who died from Alzheimer's six years ago. I decided to lighten up and move far away from this conversation.

As we continued to speak I did not understand what she was trying to say, so I responded with, "Mom, I do not understand what you just said." She must have felt a little frustrated for she answered, "If I was speaking French or Spanish, then you could not understand me." "You are absolutely correct," I said, and we both started to giggle like two teenage girls. I was thrilled, because between some things she said, there seemed to be quite a few times that she was lucid. I was able to fantasize for several moments that she did not have Alzheimer's.

I returned home almost a week now, and each day that I speak to my mom she seems to have some recollection that I was there. She cannot really express this, although she has questioned me every day as to when I will be coming to visit. Now when I exit from her home, I can no longer have my real goodbyes, for in the past she has gotten quite upset. So when I leave I simply say, "Mom, I'll see you later."

Today my mom shared with a light, upbeat voice that when she woke up she was looking all over her home for me and could not find me. For a moment it made my heart sink. It saddened me that we lived so far apart, yet there was a sound of joy that came from her voice. I knew that she was feeling happy.

Later in the day I phoned my mom again, just to hear her sweet voice. Her caregiver Trudy said that after I hung up earlier, my mom had been going around her home once again calling my name. Her voice shouted, "Lisa, Lisa, are you here?" Hearing this made my heart ache. Should I jump on a plane and run back to her?

It's been exactly one week since I was at her home.

After hanging up the phone, it left me with a piece of my heart broken in two. For the rest of day, I kept hearing Janis Joplin singing, "Take another little piece of my heart."

I often wonder how this little lady, who stands only four feet, ten inches tall, can melt my heart each day in such a way that I cannot contain my love for her. It seems to overflow with abundance and affection. Although I know that my mom cannot remember anything and may not always be able to express herself and all her feelings, I am still left with some comfort.

Deep in my heart I do feel that she is not suffering and is relatively happy. I truly believe that it is the families that suffer the most. Either way, Alzheimer's is a cruel disease that eventually takes one's life.

For me, because of my mom I have committed myself to spreading awareness about Alzheimer's and only hope that what I write can help other families find some comfort. I wish all of you much love, and I hope you know that I truly care and do understand.

COMMENTS

Lisa,

I know how you feel about your heart feeling broken. I am so happy for you, though, that you have such a sweet relationship with your mom in these difficult times. My mother became angry and unpleasant to be around in the last year. Now that Mom is gone (it's been just a little over a month), I miss her physical presence very much. I found a voice mail from her on my cell phone a couple of weeks ago where she sounded like my "real" mom and not "dementia" mom. Thankfully I saved it, because the very next day after I had it recorded it was auto-deleted from my voicemail. I hope you will always have your sweet memories of your mom, and I'm so sorry that this horrible disease is taking her from you. Mom died on August 8, and while I miss her so much I wouldn't want her to continue on the way she was.

Love,
Annabelle

———

Just as she once protected and cared for you, you now honor her by protecting and caring for her, Lisa. Thank you for sharing these experiences. They help us learn from one another by exchanging ideas.

—The Caregiver's Voice
(a virtual support group)

———

I thought about my eighty-two-year-old mother-in-law with dementia whom we love dearly. Joy sustains us as well. One thought I just had was that we live in the present more with her, since the past is disappearing. Being with her helps me appreciate the moment— flowers, clouds, scents, color. Reading your post made me feel in good company. Thanks for writing this.

—Katrina

Is My Name Lisa?

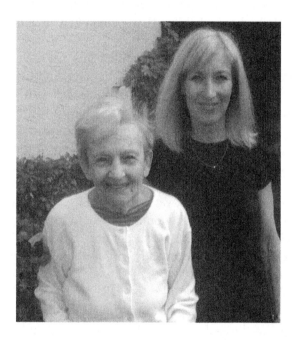

As my mom awoke in her home of twenty-four years, she exited from her bedroom and saw her caregiver Elaine sitting in her living room. Mom questioned if she was there to take care of her. Elaine answered that she was, and Mom then stated that she was hungry and wanted to know if Elaine could make her something to eat. This was a good sign, for some days she is not very hungry.

As they entered her kitchen, she wanted to know where she should sit. In some ways she has become like a young child, yet not totally. When I got to speak to her, she wanted to know when I would be visiting, and added in that she hopes I know that I could stay as long as I want.

These words that came from her lips just melted my heart. "Mom, would you like me to come and live with you?" Her answer was, "I don't think that you would really want to do that." "In that case, I have a surprise for you. Gil's coming to see you today." Mom said, "That's great, so I'll see both of you." With an upbeat tone she added in that she can hardly wait to see her kids.

I knew that I would not be seeing her for another two and a half months, yet I said nothing. I could try to explain, yet whatever I would say would not be understood and would soon be forgotten. As we continued our conversation, she quickly forgot about my brother coming to visit her.

"Mom, would you like to spell some words?" As I started our weekly exercise, starting at A and wanting to finish at Z, I asked her to spell England and then Hawaii. She stopped me on both and said, "I never heard of those words." Mom had never heard of England or Hawaii? What was going on? Can Alzheimer's have my mom's world fade to nothing? Fortunately, there were other words she did recognize enough to spell.

I realized that at this moment there was some confusion. I decided to stop spelling and tell her again that my brother was coming to visit her. "Oh, my husband is coming," she replied. "No, Mom, Gil is your son." "I know he's my son, I just call him my husband." *Okay, Mom*, I thought. *You're close but you have this backwards.*

Is there any harm if Mom thinks that my brother is her husband? I don't think so. He visits weekly, and he is the only male figure left in her life. The important part now is that she still knows who he is.

The next day when I called, I heard Elaine, her care-giver, say, "Ruth, your daughter Lisa is on the phone." This morning my mom answered with, "No, I'm Lisa." As I heard her sweet voice I giggled and I said, "Mom, I'm Lisa, so what's your name?" Mom answered with, "You tell me first." We both laughed as I said, "Okay, Mom, it doesn't matter, we can just call each other sweetheart." I thought to myself how quick and sharp her answer was. Was Mom trying to cover up her mistake or perhaps her not knowing?

Once again, it does not really matter. Mom somehow was able to understand her own confusion. So I started to serenade her with the song, "Let Me Call You Sweet-heart," and my mom joyfully joined in.

There are parts of conversations that we still can share. She has her good days and off days. I do realize that Mom is sliding backwards from Alzheimer's, yet somehow she is still able to hang in there. Her strength and her courage absolutely amazes me.

Several years ago she became my hero, and today she still can warm my heart with much joy. She brings a smile to my face. Although parts of her are now lost, I hold on tightly to all that we still can share.

COMMENTS

Another lovely, heartfelt post that has made me bite my lip to hold back some tears. I am touched by the way in which you interact with your mom on the phone. It's beautiful and inspiring.

—Jilian

Hi Lisa,

Last week was tough, but this week has been a good one for my mom, except she is being very clingy. She wants to be with me every second. She cried last night because I won't sleep with her. I have sleep issues and get anxious if I sleep in the same bed with someone. I worry I'm going to wake them because I'm very restless. I've been working with a counselor who specializes in dementia and Alzheimer's. She thinks I need to put my mom in an assisted living facility. I cried that whole day and felt so guilty. I'm going to meet with her again, and she is going to come over and observe my mom, too.

It makes me so sad. But she is getting worse, and I don't know how much longer I can do this. I give it about six months.

—Loreen

I think you sharing your journey with your mother is fantastic and helps so many people realize they aren't alone in their journey, so thank you for sharing.

—Ask My Community

Very moving post, Lisa. Brings back so many memories. Cherish your time with your mother. Love your blog!

—Katrina

Could This Be Magic?

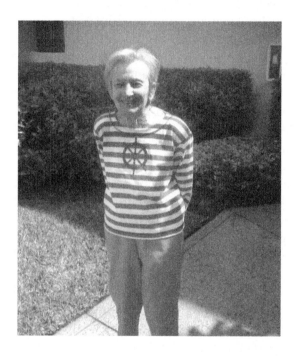

Ibelong to a support group with the Alzheimer's Association, which meets two times a month. I absolutely look forward to going there. It is a safe place to share all of my feelings with others, who I know truly understand. We all have a parent who suffers with Alzheimer's.

Yesterday while I was waiting for the bus to go to my support group, I overheard a gentlemen having a conversation with his mother. It had me reflect on how those days for me and my mom were now long gone. Like in a trance, I felt myself slipping deep into my thoughts. The days that Mom and I used to share about our lives were no longer. It left me feeling empty and sad.

I realized that this was a day that I had not yet spoken to her. I usually call her mid morning. For the last few days, I found Mom so disconnected that it was painful calling her. No sounds of laughter or joy resonated from her. Trying to get her to laugh or sing was not on the menu. She just wanted to rush me off the phone and couldn't have cared less about anything I was saying. Mom was not responsible for her actions; it was her disease reacting.

Even the conversation of asking her if I was her daughter and did she give birth to me, she answered with, "I guess so." She was able to thank me for calling, and I also got her to throw me my daily kisses. Without these kisses, my day would not be complete. I know that they will disappear, so as of now they mean the world to me. This was not one of her brighter days.

Later that evening I phoned my mom, and like magic, she and I were able to have a real conversation. She did not rush me off the phone, and there were sounds of laughter as we spoke about several different things. I knew that she was really listening, as she chirped in that she didn't want to interrupt me while I was speaking. After hanging up, I was floating on cloud nine.

The next morning she was still present, and with much conviction, she shouted how very much she loved me and wanted me to have a great day. She sounded so alive, and for several moments I could forget that she had this disease.

Two days of such clarity and she was so clear with her thinking process. How can this be? Who can understand this disease? When hearing her alive and joyful I do not question, yet when she is lost I ask myself why. Do the wires that connect in her brain connect and disconnect? When she has a day of clarity are they all connected, and when she doesn't they are disconnected? What causes several good days of joyfulness, understanding, and clarity, and then for several days she seems to slip away?

I know that the researches are trying to find a cure or even prevention for Alzheimer's. I only hope it comes in our lifetime. It's too late for my mom, yet I wonder how much they truly understand. How does Alzheimer's appear and disappear so frequently? This disease is not new for her; she has been suffering with this for at least eight years.

Yes, she has her good days and she has her not so good days. I could be flying high from the last few days, and yet I know too well how easily this magic can slip away. I think of the good moments that we still can share, even if they are less than before. So could this be magic? I do know the answer, yet my glass remains half filled not half empty. I am still grateful for whatever time we have left, and I must hold on to whenever the magic reappears.

COMMENTS

Hi Lisa,

I've found out about your blog right now. I was upset, looking for people out there who could understand. I'll be reading your pages. But what I have already noticed, reading quickly your words here and there, is that I could have written the same things myself. If only my English were better. See you soon— you and your mom.

—Julia A.

You are an inspiration, Lisa. Keep the blogs going. I am a nurse who has worked with Alzheimer's patients for the past thirty years, and you inspire me. Please add me as a friend so I can carry on reading your blog.

—Georgina

Thanks for sharing your story with us, Lisa! It really resonated with me, as I am sure it does with other adult children whose parents have Alzheimer's. Yes, this disease is quite humbling and creates "a place filled with compassion and understanding that somehow seems different than before." Well put!

—Long Island Alzheimer's Foundation (LIAF)

Thanks for that insightful experience. I was very touched. I experience this every day in my work with dementia people and their families. It never ceases to amaze me, these moments of clarity that are often so unexpected and touch my soul. I have often asked myself the same questions you asked and was hoping that someone would have responded with some sort of explanation.

—Adriane

Savoring the Moment

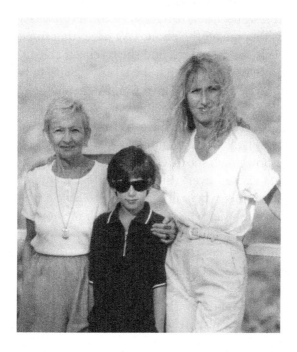

For almost a week, each day I have found my mom to be what one might say is "connected." It is true that she has absolutely no memory anymore, of the past nor the present, yet she has been sounding so refreshed and so alive.

This last week there have been no dark clouds in her life, only beautiful colors of a rainbow. Mom has been extremely happy, and her world seems to be filled with clarity. I hear the sounds of birds chirping when she answers the phone with, "Hi, sweetie." She sounds so carefree as sounds of laughter accompany her world.

We have been able to have some conversations without her rushing me off the phone. We have sung some songs and spelled some words, and she has been able to follow along with each breath that she takes. It seems to be like a miracle, as if she has escaped from Alzheimer's. We have been able to be in the moment.

Of course she is not the same mom I had before, yet this lovely lady is still my mother—a mother who can still tell me how much she loves and misses me, a mother who still gets excited every time she hears the sound of my voice, a mother who still can tell me to have a wonderful day, and a mother who still shares with me how lucky we are to have our health.

The other day after I spoke to her, I thought of my childhood and teenage years, and I thought how my mother always believed in me. I thought how supportive she was to me and how she encouraged me when I needed to hear those words from her. For some crazy reason, I took most of this for granted.

I realized today how my world has changed so drastically with our relationship. Now with every breath she takes and with the simplest of things that she may say, I hold on to each syllable that resonates from her sweet lips.

The words "I miss you and I love you" have such a deeper meaning to me. These are words that she still can speak. I realize that as time goes by, because of Alzheimer's, she may not always be able to say them. I hold on tightly and I cling to all these loving words, as if I never heard them before.

Today, until no longer, I savor all the love that I receive from her. I cherish even more, all the love that I can also give back to her. I think of this as savoring the moment, for I know all too well what probably lies ahead.

On October 21, I will be on the Walk to End Alzheimer's as a tribute to my mom, her younger brother who has passed away, and all the others who have suffered from this disease. We are all in this together and we must share in spreading awareness. We must find a cure.

COMMENTS

> Once again, your words have touched my heart. I know what you mean about taking things for granted in the past and how absolutely magical the words "I love you" can feel these days. My mom's speech was one of the first things to go, but every now and then, even in her worst moments, she will pop out a clear sentence. During those moments, when she says, "I love you," it's the best gift in the world. As far gone as she is, I have to believe that in those moments she knows what she's saying.
>
> —Anabelle

I want to wish you best of luck with your mom. Cherish, as you know from your friends, all the time you still have together. It is precious.

—Anonymous

Lisa,

It is true, our mother's teach us to value friendship. They really were our first true friends. My closest friend Debbie had a mom who suffered with Alzheimer's for years. Through her, I learned to treasure my mom even more, since you never know when this dreaded aliment takes the minds of those we love. My mom now is in the beginning stages of Alzheimer's. It so sad that their golden years get somewhat tarnished by this aliment. I wish for everyone a cure once and for all.

—Anonymous

Way to go, Lisa, for your fantastic efforts in the fight against Alzheimer's disease. I'm sure it will be a great experience, and we wish you all the best in your NYC Walk to End Alzheimer's. Good for you, and hats off to your enthusiastic efforts—we're lucky to work with people like you.

> —Amelia White, events coordinator, Alzheimer Society of Newfoundland and Labrador, Inc.

I Wonder What Mom
Is Thinking

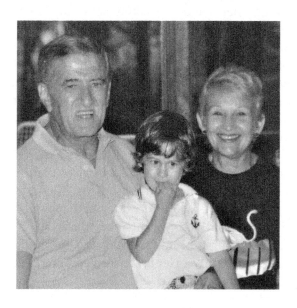

M om recently had two wonderful weeks that seemed
to abruptly come to an end. This week started off
with her sounding like she had just swallowed speed. She
was on an adrenaline rush. Mom was saying some things
that made sense and other things that I found quite difficult to understand. I wondered what was going on.

Did Mom have another urinary tract infection that
was causing her to be in what seemed like a semi-delirious

state? Probably not, since she had started an antibiotic the week before. My brother suspected that she might have had an infection. I questioned what would happen if she really needed an antibiotic. My brother Gil, being a physician, reassured me that this would not be a problem.

I found her one day speaking about my father, who passed away seventeen years ago, saying that she was waiting for him to come home from work. The next day she kept rambling on about some lady and how she remembered what had happened with her. She was making absolutely no sense at all. The next moment she was telling me that I was the best daughter in the world. Of course, I loved hearing those words.

I decided to ask her some questions to see if she, or better me, might understand. As I spoke these words, her answers were quick and responsive. "Mom, are you happy?" "Yes," she said. "I'd rather be happy and have her hold my hand." *Okay,* I thought, *who is "her"?* Then, without skipping a beat, she continued to say that she was happy to be alive. Her brain seemed to be firing and sparking all over the place.

The following day she only wanted to sleep. I'm sure this was out of total exhaustion. I only could wonder what I might find later on the other end of the phone.

Mom's journey, since she has Alzheimer's, has climbed mountains and has traveled through valleys. The rivers have flowed and at other times they have dried up. I never know what to expect. What might I experience next?

Toward the end of the week, her caregiver discovered that Mom was impacted. After she was relieved from this, she bounced back to being aware and sounding better.

Almost as if what I had experienced all week never happened. If my mom cannot tell me what is going on, how can we as caregivers know how to help them?

In a strange way this fascinates me. How does the brain connect and disconnect so quickly? I only wish that my mom could explain to me what is going on. What is she feeling? What is she thinking? Since she cannot, all that I am left with is to wonder how Alzheimer's disease can remove her vibrant ways and watch as she fades away.

Somehow, as upsetting as this can be, I have been getting used to her when she is acting this way. Yes, it hurts, and I wish I could cuddle her and take care of her, as she once did for me. Instead I take a deep breath and know in my heart that tomorrow could be a better day.

COMMENTS

Lisa,

It truly is amazing how things change minute to minute. Experiencing the disease with my mother has given me a whole new appreciation for the brain and how it works—when it works properly. It's something we all take for granted, but it's such a delicate balance. I, too, would give anything to know what thoughts are running through my mom's head at any given moment. It's such a mystery. Sending you hugs.

—Denise

───≈───

Hi Lisa:

Thank you so much for sharing this with us. Fabulous effort and fabulous blog.

—Alzheimer's Association,
Central Ohio Chapter

───≈───

I read your blog with interest, as we have just moved my mum into a nursing home in my old home town—far from where her own house was, but now near to all her grandchildren. She really doesn't remember or understand that she has moved anywhere, although she has only been there for a week—but she does wonder why there are a lot of people living with her in her house! When we explain that she is now in a nursing home where she will be properly cared for, and that she will never be on her own or lonely again, she is so happy and grateful—this, from the woman who swore she would go kicking and screaming into a home.

—Joni

───≈───

Dear Lisa,

Thank you for your blog. I just read this tonight and thought that it captures my thoughts and the love I have for my dad who has was diagnosed with Alzheimer's about five years ago. I live about six hours' drive from my parents, and my dad has been in a secure home the past three years. I phone my mom every week because I know that every day is precious and it is the least I can do when living so far away. It is now very difficult because my dad speaks very little and has largely forgotten who my family are. I wish you all the very best in your efforts to support your mom and hope that she can hold on to those memories of you her daughter for the longest time.

Kind regards,
Jonathon

Sounds of Joy

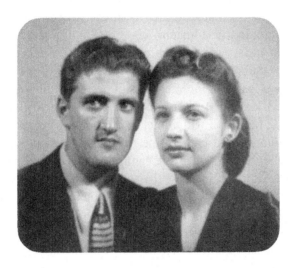

This is the second week in a row where mom has sounded really good. She has been alert, upbeat, and filled with clarity. We have been able to engage in our daily conversations. I have purchased my plane tickets to visit her and will be arriving in eight weeks. I am hoping that when I get to her home, she will still be having her better days. However, eight weeks is still a long time away.

The last time that I visited her with my husband, her days were not great and being with her was painful to watch. It brought up sadness and frustration. As my trip is getting closer, I start to feel some different emotions. As of now I am surrounded with excitement, yet feel a small knot in my stomach.

Just today, Mom so cutely said that she only hopes that she can remember when I will be arriving. She asked me to please remind her and hopes that she will not forget. I laugh with her as she speaks these words and reassure her that I will not let her forget.

Mom offered to help me make her "famous" meatloaf when I visit, since she cannot remember the recipe herself. Simple things like this excite me. I delight in each small thing she says, as if I was watching my son speak his first words or take his first steps. Her good days come and go, so I always cherish those special moments.

It doesn't matter what we may speak about, it is just that we are still able to speak. She touches my heart in so many different ways. I can no longer talk to my dad, and in reality the day will come when I can no longer speak to her.

Mom has no memory anymore of anything, including my dad, her marriage, and her youth. Maybe she still has glimpses that come to her, yet as they pass by so quickly she has no way to share them. Yet for all this she does seem happy. In her world, she does not understand the difference.

My mom and dad met when they were very young. Mom was eighteen years old when they married. Dad was only twenty one when he shipped out to serve his country. At that time mom was also pregnant with my brother.

On October 25 this year, they would have celebrated their seventieth anniversary together. My dad passed away seventeen years ago. He suffered for nine long months, while my mom traveled each and every day to see him.

I wonder how difficult it would have been for him, if he had lived, and how he would now be experiencing my mom as she drifts away. My brother and I are the only immediate family she has left.

Alzheimer's disease I believe effects the caregivers even more. We are the ones that watch how this disease destroys lives, as our loved ones lose their memory and slowly disappear. We feel the pain that they may not even realize exists.

The sounds of joy that my mom can still express are, for me, what makes me smile. She fills my heart with much joy. Every day that she still knows who I am is truly a gift to me. Mom has been so courageous, and today as always she will remain my hero.

COMMENTS

> God bless your dear mom. Cherish those shiny moments you have with your mom. I don't think there is enough awareness for caregivers. They work so hard, especially husbands, wives, or other family members or partners who are caregivers. They are so very

important. They don't seem to get any recognition for the good work they do for people with Alzheimer's.

—Ashley

Very poignant blog, Lisa. It is so hard to come to grips with the realization that one's mom may someday not know us anymore. It is a profound loss of a relationship that once was, and all loss is hard to deal with, especially one that is tied so closely with our earliest memories of who we are. It's as if we lose one of the "mirrors" in our life that serve to validate us or help us to stay grounded.

—Long Island Alzheimer's Foundation

Oh Lisa, thank you so much for sharing your mum's story. It's beautifully written and touched my heart. My mum and dad were married fifty-five years and passed away within six months of each other in 2011. They both ended up losing their lives to Alzheimer's. People said to me that they couldn't live without each other. That is something I keep in my heart, that they are together again as it should be. Take care.

—Jeannie

Lisa R. Hirsch

Hello Lisa:

My name is Mary. I am from Peru. My mother got Alzheimer's. She takes medicines like Aricept 10 mg. Quetiapine and Melatonine for sleep. Today I realized that the disease progresses. I am too sad, afraid. The next week I will take her to the doctor to check the treatment. I want to know what is the treatment your mom has. What activities does your mom do every day that keep her entertained. Kisses from Peru.

—Mary

Mom Really Melts My Heart

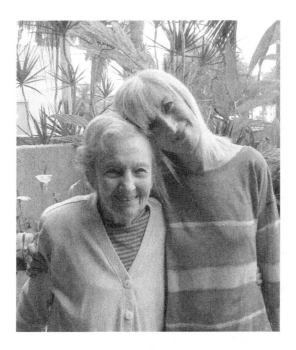

Mom and I now continuously say to each other how much we love one another. It was not always like this. It makes me wonder why when I was growing up did I not feel all this love and warmth from her? Nor did I return it. I was certainly Daddy's little girl.

I am not saying that I did not know she loved me. What I am saying is the warmth and nurturing that I felt as a child was coming from my dad, not my mom. Was it me? Was it her? Or was it both of us? My dad showed me lots of love and showered me with much affection. Could my mom had been in a crazy way jealous of our loving relationship? This I will never know or understand, and it no longer has any significance to me.

Today, and since my mom has Alzheimer's, the love we share is for me unspeakable. My mom had a good week, which left us with some amazing conversations. Every phone call ended with her asking me when I would be coming to see her. Mom would say that we have a good relationship, and the truth was, and I quote her, because she loved me more than anything in the world. She so sweetly added in that I was the best in the world, and the greatest there is.

All these words of affection and love melted my heart. It was all so magical. These are words that I can never forget. Alzheimer's has left her with no memory, yet when she still is present, she constantly shares all her love with me. Could she be making up for all the years that this was not shared ? Maybe, and certainly, yes for me.

Are we like a mirror reflecting back and forth to each other our images of love? The simple things in life that I might have once taken for granted now shine through. The words we speak each day, unless Mom is having a bad day, are filled with the brightest of sunshine. Her laugh, her smiles, her kisses now are everything to me.

At the end of each phone call, I always ask her to throw me kisses. I have shared with her that without her kisses my day would not be complete. As our last phone call came to an end, she said, "If you want your kisses, then why don't you come over, and I'll give you real kisses?" I smiled to myself knowing that I would be seeing her in six weeks, and for today she was having an exceptionally good day.

I hold so dear to my heart all our bright days, never knowing when they may fade away. Instead of thinking about the long goodbye, I focus on the long hello, and embrace all that we still can share.

COMMENTS

Hi, just wanted to say I read your blog regularly. I looked after my uncle for twelve years. He had macular degeneration and for the last five had Alzheimer's. Sadly he died in May aged eighty-six. We always joked about him getting a telegram from the queen when he was a hundred years old, a custom we have in Britain when one reaches that age, but the uncle I knew had left years before. Your mum seems such a lovely person, and I wish things could have been different for her and for you. All I can say is treasure every day. I found with my uncle there was always something he did or said that made me smile. Anyway, take care.

—Angie

Thank you for sharing the motivation and showing how Alzheimer's can be less painful
—Vanya, Beirut

I share your thoughts. I used to have dreams that my mom was suddenly back to her old self, too. It was a way of wishing that the dementia never happened, and unfortunately, one can't wish the condition away. We have to walk through the journey, rocks, bumps, potholes, and all, and hope that at the end we reach a place of understanding and compassion for others who are, or will be, traveling the same road.
—Julianne

Hi Lisa,

When I read your story of how your heart was changed towards your mom, I thought, Oh, that's me, too. When I was growing up, I didn't treat my mom too well; mostly, I ignored her. Mom moved in with me and my family (husband and two teenage boys) eight years ago. She already had dementia, but it wasn't too bad. She repeated herself and had some memory loss. Today, she has very advanced memory loss. She doesn't remember what objects are or where she is. She doesn't recognize most family members. She is still living with us. It is a challenge. I gave up my life for her along the way. I love her so much. I would do anything for her. I take it one day at a time. She is the sweetest person I know. She is happy and still signs old hymns daily. Funny how she remembers the words of old hymns like "Blessed Assurance." I will continue this path until either the Lord calls her home or she is on hospice. Thanks for sharing.

—Patricia

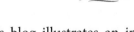

Lisa's blog illustrates an important concept when interacting with those with Alzheimer's. As Lisa succinctly says, "My mom does not remember what is true, and to me that makes no difference. At this point it does not matter. I guess what I need, or so badly want, is to delight in these cute and humorous conversations whether they make sense or not." So true, Lisa, as arguing about the accuracy of the memory of a past event only serves to upset both the person with Alzheimer's and the person who is engaged in a conversation.

It is about savoring the present, sharing the moment, and making it matter on a satisfying emotional level because after all, that is all we truly have.

—Long Island Alzheimer's Foundation

Visit Lisa's blog at www.MommyHero.blogspot.com.

CPSIA information can be obtained
at www.ICGtesting.com
Printed in the USA
LVOW04s0353071215
465713LV00022B/419/P